MW01617881

WHAT YOU MAY NOT KNOW ABOUT BARTONELLA, BABESIA, LYME DISEASE AND OTHER TICK & FLEA-BORNE INFECTIONS

IMPROVING TREATMENT SPEED, RECOVERY & PATIENT SATISFACTION

Beyond 1990's Simplistic Medicine and Its Dangerous Protocols Which are Untailored Treatment "Recipes"

Abridged Edition

James Schaller, MD, MAR

and

Kimberly Mountjoy, MS

International University Infectious Disease Press
Bank Towers • Newgate Center (Suite 305)
5150 Tamiami Trail North [Highway 41]
Naples, Florida 34103

Cover Art: Nick Botner

Lead Research and Research Study Acquisitions: Randal Blackwell

Copy Editing by Kimberly Mountjoy, Lindsay Gibson,
Jeremy Schaller and anonymous patients from all over the world

Wholesale discount requires purchase of at least twenty copies and can be in five book units. Fax request to (239) 304-1987 and (239) 263-6760.

Library of Congress Cataloging Data

Schaller, J.L; Mountjoy, K.

ISBN: 9780977397198

What you may not know about bartonella, babesia, lyme disease and other tick & flea-borne infections: improving treatment speed, recovery & patient satisfaction (abridged edition).

by J. L. Schaller and K. Mountjoy

1.Tick infections 2. Flea infections 3. Bartonella 4. Babesia 5. Lyme disease

Manufactured in the United States of America

First Abridged Edition

To my beloved friends in USA prisons,
with a hope we will end our leadership as the PRISON NATION,
especially Wayne, JD, James, Bone C., Mike and Julio,
and lead in liberty and not inmate numbers.

Let our nation return to timely trials,
end cruel and unusual excessive sentences,
allow the poor to have a good defense,
and may our peace officers never exceed the facts.

Let our prisons never have any element of torture—
the time is already a torture.

Contents

Tick and Flea Infection Emerging Medicine

Politics and Powers

I will simply be very clear and frank about the current debate over tick infections and what I see as a full-time reader and researcher. I do not mean to be disrespectful, but I do mean to start ending nonsense.

First, when you get a doctorate in medicine, you take an oath that allows you to wrestle with the complexity of medicine. Samples include dealing with emerging infections like HIV/AIDS, the new versions of Hepatitis, Stem cell technology explosions, nutritional science (which only exists outside of the pharmaceutical and medical device control of treatment options), drug resistant strains of tuberculosis, and ***over a thousand complex medical issues, so you get some room to wiggle.***

Simply, it is naive to assume the USA has all the answers when we are not even in the top 50 nations in terms of physician numbers per population, and many physicians in the United States are leaving medicine. So my comments are not meant to control over 800,000 physicians of which over 80% are not in the AMA and who care for over 300 million Americans.

I do not have all the answers in the area of tick and flea infections. And while working on my fifth book on Babesia, I found that books on parasites by smart authors have only one to three pages on Babesia; perhaps no one has all the answers.

Confusingly, the real debate or hate seems to center around the four letter word, "Lyme," referring to "Lyme disease." And the hatred this topic generates is similar to race hatred as seen in the Civil War or other periods of race hatred. Simply, this is an error, and also shows a lack of insight in how we all think.

If you trust a patient report more than an evidence based study or vice versa, I will support you. I trust both and neither.

And so in legal situations, I will defend a healer who wants to treat a patient for one infection for a short time, yet I will also support a healer who wants to treat a number of infections for a longer time. I recall a wonderful history professor, who allowed me to speak very bluntly once. I am not proud of this, but I told him he was far too hard on grading and was too confusing. He was actually a very good teacher. He simply smiled and said, “That may all be true, but when you have a doctorate, you get to present the information in a way you feel is best, and no teacher is the same, and I also get to set the line you have to cross for each grade.” He was patient. I was clueless.

And the training of the average physician is far in excess of a regular doctoral student and far more brutal, not to mention my extra college time and graduate degree. But this time allowed me to learn something pure pre-meds never learned.

IT IS IMPOSSIBLE TO HAVE COMPLETELY OBJECTIVE SCIENCE. THE SCIENTIST OR PHYSICIAN BRINGS TO THE TABLE MANY ASSUMPTIONS AND APPROACHES THAT ARE NOT SCIENCE, BUT SOCIOLOGY, PHILOSOPHIES, PREJUDICES AND MANY BIASES.

Since most pre-medicine educations are very weak on the philosophy of knowledge and of self-examination, this all sounds like fluff—but it is not fluff. Physicians must know what they bring to the table, and what guides their non-objective science and medicine. Even untrained patients are aware that physicians are biased in many ways, thus increasingly seek care outside synthetic patented pharmaceutical options and medical devices.

Those added years in humanities studies taught me to learn how to think critically and introspectively. Most physicians do not know how to weigh the assumptions and biases in every study. Simply, as

Kuhn has said in *The Structure of Scientific Revolutions,* here are some profound cliff notes about medicine. It is time for all of us to grow up and identify our religious or ultimate beliefs. For example, many years ago, anything from Harvard or the ten top journals was considered fact. This is nonsense, and I am not happy admitting to this belief, which is a type of early adolescent intellectual crush.

Some key elements on the philosophy of science are required for any basic college level understanding of science and medicine, or one is really not educated or aware of the forces creating "certainty in medicine."

Thomas S. Kuhn reminds us of what many other philosophers of science and bias have written.

A. Medical students, residents and physicians are given massive amounts of information which is a type of brain washing that may be correct in many parts, but it is a guild position. These beliefs about "facts" are required to get a medical degree and license to practice medicine. As a physician, I can assure you the volume of information is massive, uncreative, and must be deeply learned mentally to pass tests. So it has a deep hold on your mind.

B. Leaders of the medical guild can be unaware that what they hold as sacred "facts" do not fit some patients or some realities. The human body and its pathology are infinitely complex, and mastery of all aspects is impossible. Top medical sages can suppress or devalue new ideas because they undermine strongly held medical science beliefs.

C. The idea that research is unbiased is false. In fact, "research" is a strong attempt to make patients and disease fit into the positions supplied by an extremely regimented medical school and residency education. In this education you are not asked what you think, you are told what to think. Even with relentless revisions of "facts," many miss the obvious—if medical facts need to be revised routinely, perhaps "current positions" is a more accurate description for them than "facts."

D. If you present information that challenges the positions of the core medical community, you are treated like an anarchist, hated and degraded when new, possibly contradictory information emerges. It is threatening the core beliefs of the medical community "guild"—since they believe the current position is just fine. The nucleus members of the guild holding to these principles use their journals, professional societies, continuing education classes and mentoring to preserve the past core beliefs.

I am currently writing an updated tick and flea infection text to help the many fine healers and patients seeking the most up to date knowledge and the best tailored care. It contains over 400 pages of references alone. Below is a small sample of the points from this textbook. When one studies emerging infections, it is impossible to finish learning. I continually update my positions every season.

I stand on the shoulders of at least 500 authors and medical professionals, and while I might not always agree with their positions, they push you to find critical new information.

It should be noted that a negative finding, such as the discovery that a certain type of treatment fails, is always very useful. A poor treatment leads to increased illness over time, even if in the initial months it appears to be useful.

Please consider these points below. My goal is not to have you agree 100%, but to have you simply ponder these issues.

What do we do with people who still feel ill after a treatment with doxycycline at the approved dose?

When a person has "Lyme disease," is there ever a reason to treat longer than a few weeks? If the treatment is helping the patient more each week, do you still stop treatment at a set time? In other words, if Jane is better in her function, or some sign or symptom each week, do you still stop at a set day?

As a Former Director of a Research Center in Infectious Disease has said, "No one is saying that they're not suffering from something. It's just that it doesn't have anything to do with chronic Lyme disease."

Let us start with what is fairly obvious in some unknown percentage of patients. Simply, they do not feel well, and while they may have some psychiatric or cognitive complaints, they do not meet criteria of somatization or hypochondriasis, because *when I do testing for things like inflammation markers, and anti-inflammation hormones or peptides, nutrient deficits, hormone status, etc., I see pathology that is medical, not PRIMARY psychiatric disorders*.

It is important that we accept that some percentage of patients remain ill regardless of the approach. And I do not think at this stage it matters if it is 5% or 95%. If it is you or your loved ones, 5% is worth serious discussion, meaning, are you going to stop care if your relative is getting better on any treatment?

Few physicians always use probiotics with antibiotics. And those that do prescribe them do not understand 99% of probiotics are very poor.

Fifteen years ago I clung to a few preferred probiotics, due to the usual seduction—many strains at high colony numbers. I had health care workers take high doses of these probiotics, after which they stopped for 5 days and I did a stool culture. Every stool sample yielded the same result: a total lack of the good bacteria required for health. These brands would not prevent a C. difficile bacterial infection of the intestines—a real problem. No one should ever be given an antibiotic for any duration, 2 weeks or 2 months, without top probiotics. I mention this in more detail in my first Babesia textbook, *The Diagnosis and Treatment of Babesia*. Simply, if no number or other further designation follows the name of the bacteria, it is a strain with no proof it can bind and proliferate in the 30 feet of intestine. Also, having only one strain of good bacteria is like having one finger. Some of this information was available in the 1980's.

Some probiotics with no specified strains have been used in research to decrease intestinal disease. For example, they merely refer to an "acidophilus." I would see these as possibly of use since in a study of patients in the real world they appear to offer a benefit, even though they may have sub-optimal strains. Only about a dozen international probiotics are known to bind to the gut wall, reproduce rapidly and work together like a piano player's fingers. Two good ones are Theralac and Dr. Ohhira probiotics.

In summary, I would suggest ***antibiotics never be used without top quality carefully selected probiotics***—the duration of antibiotic use does not matter. There is always some unknown risk.

If physicians are sincerely concerned about C. difficile and resistant strains, they should start by reading *Probiotics: A Clinical Guide,* by Floch and Kim, who are both physicians.

Always start one treatment at a time, and do not add or increase two things in the same day.

Years ago the chairman of a famous Ivy League medical department and the editor of the top pediatric journal asked me to write on dosing medication to decrease side effects. All treatment of any kind needs to be isolated. You should typically add only one new treatment at a time, and no more than one new thing in a day. Further, if you increase a dose, it is regarded as a **new** treatment. Therefore, if you start three things and do not feel right, get a rash or cannot work because of the treatment, you have no idea how to tailor it. Why? You have three possible causes for your problem. Being told to "grin and bear it" is not very caring and it is not tailored care. If we can tailor a suit, we can tailor biochemical interventions.

The suggested testing using only a direct Lyme ELISA test is confusing.

The ELISA test is respected lab testing, but while it is very good in some situations, tick and flea infection medicine may not be one of them. For example, patients can have a marked change in results by simply being 35,000 feet high in a plane, having a surgery or for many other reasons. But even if 90% are correct, that means 1 in 10 will be missed. Since the infections carried by the Ixodes tick may be serious if untreated, this is a risk, assuming even a 90% sensitive ELISA test result.

What do you do when the ELISA changes from positive to negative (or vice versa) without any medical intervention? As I said, diagnosis is messy in emerging infections, and that is reality. In order for physicians to keep their insurance contract, they have to order the least number of tests possible—it is like a source of pride and skill. Amusingly, medical board members, appointed as a reward for involvement in political medicine, are acting for insurance companies by an excessive dependence on one lab test to diagnose, and by often calling more complete lab testing which shows positive findings "wasted labs" and "bad medicine."

If it is good enough for MAYO, HOPKINS, and the CLEVELAND CLINIC, it is surely good enough for any passionate clinician who wants to do a good and thorough job. No one would dare attack an Ivy League physician for ordering extra labs.

Let me make this simple. You have a parent, spouse, sibling or child who is ill. Seven smart physicians are unable to find the cause of their sickness. So you go to see a specialist in diagnostic medicine.

This doctor wants to order ten tests that have never been ordered before. Indeed, the lab staff and your primary care doctor have no idea what these tests are meant to show. Do you do these unfamiliar labs or ignore the consult? Your loved one's health is hanging in the balance.

Do not be more "moral" than the DEA if you need controlled drugs to function.

Some patients need strong treatments to keep their job or function in school. These may include medicines for sleep, anxiety, focus, pain or depression. Some options are traditional medications that are controlled substances. These can all be made into transdermal treatments, or treatments that go through the skin. Some may reject these as "unnatural" perhaps because they have not been used carefully since some healers do not understand that in ***an infected or inflamed brain these medications cannot be dosed in "routine suggested ways."***

If a patient has depression, restlessness and trouble with concentration, do you know which of these should be handled first? I strongly suggest depression is always treated before anxiety, and anxiety before focus defects. If you do not do this carefully and with close communication between the patient and the healer, you can commit chemical battery.

Other options for depression, anxiety, focus or pain may be called "functional, integrative or alternative medicine." Some of these are very effective, but can fail with neurological infection or brain inflammation. For example, SAM-e is an exceptional anti-depressant, but St. Johns Wort is normally ineffective in serious depression. No single school of medicine has all the answers. Therefore, my appeal is to be open to what works. "Natural" options are often profoundly useful. However, in some areas we have very limited natural options, and I am not going to lie to a patient and oversell an alternative medicine option that usually is ineffective. Some health care workers are excited about one type of treatment. I am excited when Mrs. Jones or Mr. Smith experience help from a wide range of possible treatments, and the labs show the treatment is actually working. Each patient comes before any type of pet treatment.

Medicine is dead without both the freedom of thought and the ability to treat patients individually.

Much medical care is reduced to being a bank teller or lawn mower repairman. Further, the ability to see uniqueness in each patient, and not merely trends, makes medicine both human and advanced. Why? Because the biochemistry of infections and unique human bodies create the possibility of profound variety in treatments.

Freedom of Thought in the French Tradition is useful here. I am the son of a genius physician father who served with both the American Army and Navy. This meant I was born in my beloved France while he served, and I mention this only because **the French can teach us a lesson on intellectual freedom.**

Watch two men in passionate and sober debate in a French café. Minutes later they are eating and enjoying that special treasure of friendship exemplified by the second US President John Adams and his best friend and wife, Abigail Adams, or as depicted in the Hebrew Bible between Jonathan and David.

My point?

Many French people ***do not fuse an idea with the person holding to that opinion, and once discussed, it is shelved.*** In other countries, you ***are*** your opinion. Amazingly, you can be the sports team you praise. This needs to be very clear when one is dealing with beliefs in the area of emerging flea and tick infections with new species found monthly. We need to make our point passionately and reasonably but without reaching the point of hatred. When people reach that place, they do unethical, unnecessary and destructive things to the physicians who disagree with them. As an MD, I can offer an opinion and feel that it is as good as yours, unless you are--by actual study and actual experience--better than me. Infectious disease experts are typically not experts on tick and flea infections, since they do not have the time to read 7,000 journal articles while working full-time with HIV, Herpes, MRSA, Hepatitis and the other top ten infections. In the same way, I will never do surgical work because that requires supervised cutting skills that I have never learned.

Further, patients and researchers filter. Those who are of the Lyme only infection model go to those who hold to that approach. And if they get very ill later, they never go back. Others see physicians who are very IV centered and use the HIV or TB model. They believe the long-term IV Lyme centered model is the best approach.

Each of them sees the annoyed patients of the other, but not the successes. I know patients that have gone to IDSA physicians who were treated 30 days or less and have been fine for at least five years. I have seen patients who were treated exactly according to IDSA guidelines yet were still very ill. And they are becoming disabled. The issue is not why they are worse, since it is not always an IV antibiotic deficit, but simply the reality that the patient is not functioning after "curative care." And let us not mention they need psychiatric medicines for their residual body troubles. All tick-borne infections can cause neurologic and psychiatric troubles.

In this book I will discuss things definitely not known by most specialists in infectious disease or those with a serious interest in Flea and Tick infections.

Further, even I do not agree with my positions after six months, because so much is changing and new in every aspect of these bacteria, protozoa and viruses. Emerging infections and a set "guideline" kept over five years may be a functional contradiction. "Emerging" and a single type of treatment does not make sense logically or practically.

If you do not agree with what I write on a topic, fine. I might agree I was wrong next year.

Some feel "correctness" is based on location of the physician's office or what staff they have joined. Having rejected prestigious places repeatedly, I do not get this medical Mecca or Vatican type of thinking.

My father went to a highly respected Ivy League Medical school. I rejected invitations to the same school, in order to avoid being mugged and shot, and because he was not pleased with his experience. Sites that rate schools are silly, because faculty can change in a year, and very few in the USA have the advanced wisdom and time to know each aspect of a training program.

So I do not weigh the expertise of any physician based on the name of an institution. Some with my temperament are adverse to required "meetings" because they can waste time. Some select physicians are as passionate about study as any person running a large grant study. Yet some reading oriented physicians also want to actually see patients, get to know them, and offer advanced personal tailored medical care based on both published materials and consults with many solid state, national, and international clinicians.

Indeed, one of my close friends, who spent much time at the National Institutes of Health and was part of many large studies, is now a strong clinical research practitioner, and the pearls he has found from treating patients he shares with me one to ten years before a study confirms his experience with hundreds. This type of physician is a legitimate practitioner, and saying one has to do either pure "research" or pure "clinical" care is too polarized.

Indeed, a functional cancer cure and other discoveries I have made occurred after patients went to the top respected medical centers in America, and were not helped. In my training in medicine and metaphysics, we were taught how to think, weight the studies, and that clinical medicine often had no study to use or available studies had so many exclusion criteria that generalized use was difficult. "Pure patients" with one issue really do not exist, and likely never in those with one or more tick bites over years.

I have a strong belief that a doctorate in medicine allows one some freedom to seek out options to heal. These treatment proposals should not be limited by large insurance companies or pharmaceutical companies defining the options in our tool box. Simply, if a physician and a competent patient want to pursue a particular treatment, as long as it is not a profound and clear danger to the patient, they should be allowed to make that choice.

Therefore, I do not regard doctors as children, so I will defend, by all ethical and aggressive means, any attack on any position regarding the treatment of tick and flea-borne infections. I will defend any sincere practitioner regardless of their style of treatment. Since I have yet to meet someone who has been reading research papers full-time on these infections for eight years, I have no one that I feel fully shares my identical opinion. So I would support those who reject some of my beliefs on these emerging infections.

Why? Thankfully, we do not have Stalins or Hitlers in medicine. We have patients, and more new and emerging information on these infections than any human can read. Deferring to a small number of "top studies" or to "patient experiences" is not definitive medicine. It is an assumption about knowledge showing a lack of philosophical maturity common in those who have had rigorous science training divorced from advanced modern philosophy. It is perfectly fine if you do not agree with each new very specific clinical real world medical point that I make. I do not even agree with many of my own practices nine months ago in this area of tick and flea infections.

I believe very strongly in liberty, therefore, I do not believe that doctors who have soberly reflected on their treatment approach should ever be sued or reported to medical boards. States are coming to the same conclusion.

The lesson of the debates in New York State, in which a widely known MD asserted that the duration of one infection--Lyme--can be flexible, is that making every doctor treat every patient for a short time or for a long time is outside the law of medicine.

When a physician studies intensely, and for many years, in one area of medicine they slowly develop a strong advanced set of research based beliefs. While this approach can drop their yearly income markedly, if they read over 15 hours a week, it will profoundly lift their wisdom in any topic. Reading 40-50 hours a week has allowed me to offer a very small number of patients very thorough care.

Bartonella is no footnote and is more common than Lyme.

Many years ago when I first got involved in the **super specialty** of tick and flea infection medicine, no one took Bartonella seriously. It was presented as an easy to kill infection, and of no real concern. It was rarely discussed at infection medicine meetings, in guidelines or infection textbooks. (I noticed the same thing after publishing four books on Babesia--the parasite books I purchased only had two pages on this serious infection).

When I published the most recent book on Bartonella, it showed that Bartonella did not have two or three skin patterns, but vast numbers. This was a fully new and massively expanded diagnostic tool based on reading the world literature and examining heavily infected patients. I was also surprised that no one was looking for the chemicals altered by the presence of Bartonella and the dynamic of these chemicals when both Babesia and Bartonella are present. You can read this in the latter sections of my textbook, *Babesia 2009 Update*.

This year a new human Bartonella species was added to the over thirty-five Bartonella species publically published in Genetic Data banks. It was discovered and highlighted by the talented veterinarian researcher Edward Breitschwerdt. He has said things more clearly than the ideas I was pondering in 2005, while doing most of my Bartonella book reading. He has said simply, but with devastating and highly useful clarity that **Bartonella testing is terrible, the treatments are poor,** it is typically found on the outside of red blood cells, and the current research on Bartonella is pathetic—one study at NIH. If this was not enough, he said in 2011, **"Bartonella is carried by more vectors than any infection on the earth."** So it is hardly a backdoor "co-infection." Indeed, this month Bartonella was literally shown to alter human DNA. The implications of this possibility are staggering, and may support what I reported six years ago—Bartonella is not killed simply or easily. My appeal is simple: treating it like a footnote infection is outdated and harmful.

Finally, based on the position above that Bartonella has the largest number of vectors in nature, perhaps Lyme is the "co-infection."

The treatments for Bartonella are based on terribly outdated testing or are very experimental without real proof by *indirect* and advanced direct testing.

I am embarrassed to admit that six years ago I felt you could rule out Bartonella by a simple antibody test—an IgM and an IgG. When only one species was being tested for in North America, it was also easy to ignore that other Bartonella species infect humans. Further, in 2005 I was amazed to learn how much Bartonella suppresses immunity. It lowers fevers and at times drops antibodies for many common tick and flea-borne infections. Further, we found that most proposed treatments in traditional and integrative medicine at best stun Bartonella, and do not cure or even drop body load much. Treatments that are promoted because patients "feel better" are not clear proof. Patients feel better for a hundred reasons, and that is not science, it is psychotherapy. Many healers treating Bartonella are using good treatment options, but they do not know how to use indirect and direct testing to confirm effectiveness. This means treatment variables are chaotic, and at times treatments are mixed up like a stew. This approach is very dangerous because Bartonella can cause literal death, in addition to injuring every organ twenty different ways (based on a review of the world literature).

If someone has a Western Blot with a "band" or antibody highly specific against Lyme, how can that be ignored?

The interpretation of the Lyme Western Blot test is very faith based, and is not like pure math. Indeed, in one recent study from China, they take the position that one band or antibody against an infection shows the infection is present. They even consider the non-specific spirochete antibody to be useful if you prove it is not caused by other spirochetes.

Let us talk about how to interpret a Western Blot test. Some say these tests are either "negative" or "positive." This does not sound like medicine, but an arbitrary religious-type faith position.

If a person has one "fingerprint band," some feel this is proof of Lyme disease. These highly specific bands, widely accepted in the world literature, are 13, 14, 17, 21, 23, 24, 25, 28, 31, 34, 35, 37, 39, 47, 50, 54, 83, 84, 93 and 94. The lab can be a junk lab that invests nothing to optimize their testing kit, but if one of these bands is positive—Lyme is present. In the last six years IGeneX has been attacked for their Western Blot despite the fact that five samples every four months from New York State have been correct 98% of the time for over a decade. What lab is that correct on negative and positive blind controls?

Has any other lab invested so much for so long, to create the best test? If your clinician wants to use an ELISA first, this is a gamble. To put it bluntly, many patients and physicians report that the ELISA test as a screening tool is useless, missing even the most obvious PCR positive patients with clear past histories of massive Bull's Eye rashes, which, while not the norm, provide evidence of spirochetes. Do we assume all patients reporting a clear tick bite and many tick infection symptoms are 100% liars or inept?

The best treatment for you is not merely one intervention type or school of healing.

You should never be treated by only one school or philosophy of healing or only one type of intervention. Too many healers are only using the options that are rooted in their highly specific training.

The treatment of tick infections involves many types of medicine and affects many body systems. Therefore healers need to know many types of medicine. Many types of healing can be of use. But I also believe in each school of healing some parts are not of use in treating tick and flea-borne infections. One reason I have had to learn so many types of medicine over the last two decades is that my education was obviously only a starting point as a healer. I have had to try so many credible treatments of different types because that offered the best help to patients. No one type of treatment works for all the facets of tick and flea-borne infections. One has to have a broad range of options.

Treatment given season after season and year after year with poor monitoring might be cheap, but it is very inadequate care.

Currently I drive the cheapest car I could find. If a huge SUV hits me, I am toast. What is the point of the illustration? You get what you pay for. If someone is seeing 20 or more patients a day, that is hardly going to allow them to adjust and tune many facets of your treatment. Tick infections hit virtually every part of the body. So a healer has to know many systems of the body—hormones, inflammation, nutrients, improving functionality quickly, compounding medicine, preventing cancer and preventing clots. Further, they must also understand that these infections can impact any organ or human body chemical system.

The bite you see is rarely the first bite.

While it is well known that the more common stages of biting ticks are very hard to see, what is not appreciated is that, **based on animal studies, any rash may be a sign of a past bite** that occurred 1, 5, or 20 years earlier. Further, more advanced and informed lab tests, showing the biochemical domino effect of tick infections over years, are often very abnormal in people reporting symptoms from a "first bite." If you are a physician or nurse practitioner and do not know the 15-20 indirect labs altered by tick and flea infections, that is a concern.

The diagnosis of tick and flea infections is dirty, confusing and hardly easy.

For example, what do you think when the Lyme ELISA is negative, only the IgG 23 "fingerprint" Lyme infection band on the Western Blot is positive, and a PCR for Lyme is positive?

That does not fit some formulas proposed in emerging infection medicine. Further, in traditional medicine, a diagnosis is made by an excellent history and interview of the patient followed by a physical exam—labs merely support the diagnosis. That is one reason I noted the dermatology differences in vast numbers of highly infected Bartonella patients compared to uninfected normal patients. Bartonella alters blood vessels and skin tissue in perhaps over eighty skin markings. When I started my investigation of vast numbers of published and unpublished skin signs, only two or three patterns were discussed. Now, slowly, people are mentioning and posting images of Bartonella that have never existed as "Bartonella images" in the 100 years since its discovery.

The new wave of Lyme disease or Babesia infection mockery is both naive and unkind to patients.

Tick infections are emerging infections. Emerging means no one has the foundation to be cocky. Some believe physicians are only useful when they "reassure" patients they do not have any of the hundred possible species and variants of the infectious agents carried in an Ixodes tick. Since more and more of the population is moving away from traditional allopathic (MD) medicine, perhaps this is not a good issue to mock. One can suggest a course of action for any infection if they wish. But the notion of utter mastery shows a lack of insight into the many complex ways these infection clusters exist after a few bites by the Ixodes tick over a few years. Amusingly, one researcher mentioned to me she found tapeworm DNA in an Ixodes tick. I do not think she or I feel you can get a tapeworm from a tick bite, but if you can find tapeworm DNA inside the gut of a tick, you can find virtually anything.

The loss of insight and an increase in rigidity is sometimes the first symptom of infection with brain and body inflammation.

One danger in some people is they have no idea they are losing productivity or insight, because that awareness comes from the higher and more advanced areas of the brain. Self-reflection is an advanced type of brain function, and it can be impaired if more than a small area of the brain is infected and inflamed. Once someone has this problem they may never be willing to be examined.

Chronic tick infections over years drop anti-inflammation chemicals and increase inflammation chemicals with serious results.

When one's body is chronically inflamed, some other things start to happen. One's vulnerability to autoimmunity increases and depending on which type of autoimmunity, one can become disabled or die. Further, one can have an increase in allergies. These can be allergies to foods, synthetic medicines, and at times even herbs. Finally, one can also become highly sensitive to volatile chemicals, and it requires immense work to maintain a work, school or living location free of synthetic chemicals.

Routine treatments to reverse systemic and deeply entrenched inflammation are generally trivial and ineffective.

If you read a book on lowering inflammation, you will see the same twenty options that are listed in other books or journal articles. Unfortunately these do not work when dealing with immense long term chronic inflammation secondary to a series of missed tick and flea-borne infections. We have some options for this problem, but they are outside the realm of this short article.

The dose that causes misery is not required for effective killing.

Some healers feel you should never feel an effective antibiotic, and others feel you are not getting any benefit unless you feel terrible. As the Greeks and Calvin said, perhaps the best position is the middle way. If a medication seems to be having an effect that causes discomfort which is not a side effect, what is wrong with lowering it to a dose just below the level of discomfort? I am almost embarrassed to raise this issue, but do so because it is a common issue.

Very advanced pharmacology is needed to address physical, neurologic, hormonal, nutritional and psychiatric problems in tick infection medicine.

Sometimes the most important first treatments are not things that kill infections. Sometimes people need care for their extremely low vitamin D level, depression, irritability, anxiety, rage, fatigue, insomnia, cognitive deficits and agitation which are hardly rare with tick and flea infections left untreated for a significant period of time.

This is very important and few physicians are familiar with the dosing for these infections and the common presence of inflammation in the brain which causes these problems. For example, we suggest all capsules and tablets should never be started over the quarter mark of the smallest option. But the end effective dose may be profoundly high. These are not primary psychiatric disorders, but disorders secondary to infections, infection debris and inflammation of the brain.

The notion that an Ixodes tick carries only "Lyme Disease" is a 1990's notion.

If a clinician uses advanced, direct and highly important indirect testing to look for the increasing number of infections carried by tiny Ixodes ticks (deer ticks), it is clear that organisms besides Lyme are present routinely in Ixodes ticks. The idea that Ixodes ticks only carry one infection is a disaster. Ixodes ticks carry multiple bacteria, parasites, and viruses. For example, Bartonella is far more common than Lyme disease.

There is no correct starting dose for virtually any medication.

I was asked years ago by two top editors to write an article on "sensitive and careful dosing in clinical practice." They noticed within my various papers we were pointing out the need for tailored dosing instead of chemical battery. For example, all medications should begin with a first dose that is below a full tablet or capsule, because sometimes it is 20 times more effective than normal. Always start with a fraction of the lowest dose pill and this can be increased over a mere 24 hours.

One should never increase or start two treatments on the same day.

This is chaos, and causes confusion if you have a reaction to the medications. You do not know if one of the treatments is creating a side effect or is working well. Also, if a patient develops uncomfortable feelings, either from the die off of an organism or from medication side effects, they become demoralized, and the cause is unclear with many treatments. Simply, no two people have even been treated by me the same from start to finish, and this is why a cure book on all major tick-borne infections cannot be published.

Further, if you increase one treatment and add another, you have implemented two new treatments on the same day. I would not do this if it can be avoided.

Is the new explosion of "Lyme Literate" or "LLMD experts" really trained to do more than basic screening?

Generally when I am trying to pursue an expertise in any aspect of tick and flea-borne infections, I spend years engaged in full-time reading on the topic and try to talk with the leaders around the world who know the most on the topic. Unfortunately, as of 2010, "Lyme Literate" really means that you have gone to a couple conferences, learned the basics from the last five to ten years, and some also shadowed one or two physicians for days to a week while they see patients.

This is a good starting place, but does not make one "tick-infection literate" in any serious manner. Finding someone that knows how to use a wide range of labs which will check for a direct and indirect presence of the infections from ticks, who has read thousands of articles, and consults with physicians and scientists regularly for success and failures along with finding new solutions is extremely rare in the world. Yet we do need every screening healer we can get.

Routine speed I.V. treatment of most new patients is an error.

Some individuals treating Lyme disease do a fairly rapid assessment and quickly put all of their patients on an I.V. like they are running a mill. It is almost as if they say "It is nice to meet you, let's get you started on your I.V. quickly." There are many problems with this approach and far too many to discuss here. The first problem is that the volume of spirochetes that can die with an invasive I.V. could be too much and release Lyme debris and/or Lyme biotoxins, such as BbTox1, which can increase inflammation.

I.V. and all other types of Lyme treatment work profoundly better if one or more new Bartonella treatments are used. We find these new treatments every few seasons. As previously stated in my first Townsend article on the "Reasons for Lyme Treatment Failure," the most common treatments for Bartonella come from a mere 25 basic Bartonella treatment articles or infection handbooks. They lead to relapse even when they appear to work for variable periods of time.

I.V. gall bladder emergencies are too frequent. One reason some insurance companies do not want to do prolonged I.V. treatment is because of gallbladder emergencies. I am fairly stunned that the only thing given to protect the gall bladder and liver with the use of I.V. medications is Actigall, and some do not prescribe anything when giving I.V. treatment. Many have little knowledge of advanced ways to protect the liver, and yet use liver stressing treatments. For example, any dose of azithromycin, Mepron, Malarone, Diflucan or I.V. or injected muscle antibiotics can stress the liver, and low doses that do not stress the liver may lead to residual infections.

Following the guidelines of practitioners with famous names, university titles or organization leadership positions might be unwise.

If a healer is famous or has a title or "chair" or is high in an organization, the more brutally busy the healer can be, sometimes working 12 hours virtually every day. So this hcaler can never read high volumes of new material published this season. Therefore, no organization, government agency, web site or person has the definitive, updated information on tick-infection medicine in the USA or the world. No single organization or group of organizations can provide people with authoritative instruction in how to treat each individual profoundly unique patient.

All guidelines for medicine are flawed and outdated within one month of publication.

The explosion of new published material and non-published discoveries by hundreds of international healers makes guidelines mere suggestions.

Hundreds of thousands of articles are published every few months. In our practice, we have only published five percent of what we have found. Similarly, many fellow researchers I know also have limited time to publish their discoveries.

Further, as mentioned before, the great philosopher of science, Kuhn, has shown that there are so many variables that impact all scientists, that the notion that any group of physicians can give unbiased purely scientific recommendations is impossible. Obvious guideline errors are present in all current tick and flea-borne infection guidelines.

Different guidelines have unusually specific treatment plans which are not even appropriate for cars from the 1950s, let alone current automobiles which have different types of oil and different amounts of recommended oil, and electrical and computer systems that are stunning in complexity.

The human body, when it is infected with a cluster of tick infections, is a billion times more complex than any automobile. Some guidelines use highly dated doses from studies that are fifteen years old. Other guidelines do not even mention infections such as persistent human atypical Bartonella, which has vastly more vectors than Lyme disease, or Babesia which suppresses the immune system in highly specific ways that some guideline agencies and groups seem to totally ignore.

In conclusion, one example that months matter in research relates to the CDC Morgellons' study which admits it intentionally ignored critical indirect Bartonella tests TNF-alpha and IL-6, and used highly insensitive markers for inflammation (sedimentation rate). They opted for a “skin-primary” approach, which I have said repeatedly over five years is a waste of time. They also seemed to limit the importance of fatigue and cognitive deficits which are not associated with delusions.

What is not mentioned in the CDC paper is a new paper by Middelveen and Stricker, showing spirochetes cause colored fibers in bovines as part of their full-body disease--my Morgellons’ patients always have full-body issues. Clearly, this paper was not read in the months before the CDC paper hit the world news. So months matter in clinical real-world medicine.

Sample References

Pearson ML, Selby JV, Katz KA, Cantrell V, Braden CR, et al. (2012) Clinical, Epidemiologic, Histopathologic and Molecular Features of an Unexplained Dermopathy. PLoS ONE 7(1): e29908. doi:10.1371/journal.pone.0029908

Middelveen, M., & Stricker, R. (2011). Clinical,Cosmetic and Investigational Dermatology,4,167-177

Savely, V., Stricker, R. (2010). Morgellons disease: Analysis of a population with clinically confirmed microscopic subcutaneous fibers of unknown etiology. Clinical, Cosmetic and Investigational Dermatology 3, 67–78.

Evans NJ, Blowey RW, Timofte D, et al. Association between bovine digital dermatitis treponemes and a range of ‘non-healing’ bovine hoof disorders. Vet Rec. 2011 Feb 26;168(8):214. Epub 2011 Feb 15.

A complete lack of meaningful knowledge of the immense magnitude and danger of Bartonella is very dangerous.

This stealth bacterium has over ten different ways to infect you, and not merely a few types of ticks. It kills, harms every organ, decreases fevers and immune defenses, and does not fully respond to the top ten "published" traditional or alternative treatments. In one case report it appears that Bartonella turned off all the antibodies to five tick-borne infections, including its own antibody titer levels. In this medical family they self-treated with a new Bartonella agent and this resulted in an explosion of western blot Lyme disease bands and all major deer tick infection antibody titers suddenly rose to profound levels because the immune system was no longer suppressed against them by Bartonella. Therefore, merely by the use of this newly uncovered Bartonella treatment, all of these patients' negative labs at a large national lab turned positive after being repeatedly negative.

The use of fetish, "favorite" medications, herbs or newly "discovered" causes of prolonged illness can waste time for patients.

Of course, any healer studying traditional or progressive medications is serving all. My appeal in this criticism is not to reject the fine work done by at least two hundred people internationally on traditional antibiotics, protozoa medications, anti-viral drugs, herbs used for a wide range of infections, essential oils, and at least fifty progressive alternative treatments.

However, like the experience of falling in love, when one love becomes all you think about, this is not optimal medicine when you fall in love with a few treatments.

For example, minocycline, tetracycline, clarithromycin, rifampin, azithromycin, HBOT, Rife, special saunas, ozone, I.V. nutrients to "boost immunity," chelation, confused detox formulas, Artemisia derivatives, essential oil combinations, I.V. medications, various weak alcohol based herbal programs, various energy machines, and a hundred other options found in chat rooms and Lyme disease "information" sites, are not meant to be the sole or primary style of all patient treatment.

Carpenters use select tools at select times for select needs. Nevertheless, with my thanks for the above passion of those that promote these and hundreds of others of treatments, they have to pass blind rigorous simple direct and indirect testing to show they work, and very few know how to do such testing. I feel it is an error to only use an antibiotic which has limited mechanisms for killing bacteria.

I have published the most current textbook on Artemisia derivatives, including artemisinin (qinghaosu) and many other toxic forms that should be avoided. And yet, despite being the most recent practical clinical book on the topic, based on a year of full-time study with Chinese consultants and WHO consultants, it has been ignored, and instead of artesunate being used, inferior artemisinin is used. Why?

The final approach that is worthy of mention is the "I only do natural treatments" approach.

Unfortunately when I interview some of these individuals, many of whom are quite smart and well read, they are aware of allopathic medication side effects, but not the toxic components of the herbs they are using. Individuals using essential oils, including those that prescribe them, usually have never read a book on the various toxicities and safety concerns of essential oils. Some of them have excellent effects and others can provide help, but also have side effect risks and others should never be used internally at all in anything more than a minimal dose.

The "new" yearly or bi-yearly cause of Lyme disease treatment failures is possibly wrong.

A few years ago, the existence of a Lyme biofilm was proposed. Many spirochetes make biofilms so this was not really a surprise, but not addressing these may undermine treatment outcomes.

Indeed, many types of spirochetes in the mouth are known to cause biofilms, and they are believed to limit antibiotic effectiveness. Organizations with millions in grants and research money have never addressed this issue.

I am currently working on a textbook that addresses the many treatment options for attacking biofilms. No article or book exists that explores the twenty-plus ways that I would propose to beat a Lyme biofilm. It is believed by some professionals that highly specific enzymes, drugs, or one mineral can undermine a Lyme biofilm. Yet enzymes are like highly specific keys, and no single enzyme has been a proven "key" to undermining a Lyme biofilm.

I was appreciative that a few brilliant researchers found that the Bb Lyme spirochete had a biofilm in recent years. But I was actually stunned this was felt to be new, since spirochetes routinely have biofilms, and there is immense research on dental spirochetes going back many years on biofilm promoting dental disease. A review of the major world literature shows about 25 treatment options to handle biofilms. No one has offered more than a small number of basic options to beat this problem. Perhaps it increases treatment relapses and failures, but that is not what I usually see.

If biofilms slow treatment, here are a few sample options from the 25 in the literature. NAC is a liver health supplement given for acetaminophen overdose (Tylenol) and it undermines some biofilms.

Another approach is to give a constant select antibiotic, such as azithromycin (Zithromax), and over time if the blood level is constant, it will connect to the surface of the biofilms and work its way into the biofilm, and ultimately into contact with the bacteria. Finally, digestive enzymes such as proteases are sometimes able to hinder many biofilms. Some promote a single enzyme as the magic cure to every biofilm type and variation made by tick and flea based infections. My strong opinion is these are never the reason for relapse alone, and one enzyme is never a sure thing against the many types of biofilms in humans.

Is it wise to reject a consult with a top thought leader due to cost?

When I think back over the hundreds of physicians, PhDs, herbal experts, nurses, alternative healing practitioners and even poorly educated addicts whom I treated decades ago, it is clear to me that, while none of them was perfect, all have helped me immeasurably. Currently, at least 50 physicians are defamed for their fees when treating tick-borne infections and this can end their entire career. Many physicians who are associated with the Infectious Diseases Society of America (IDSA) have said that patients with tick infections are harder to deal with than those with other very serious infections. Some physicians stop their treatment of any patients with tick or flea infections because of the way they are treated.

The same applies to bonding with a healer. I often seek the wisdom of people that may be annoying, irritable, tired, simplistic, insulting, or confusing. But the fact of the matter is that virtually every healer I have known, regardless of specialty, philosophy and ideology, has taught me a lesson that helps patients. I have literally seen patients decide to go with physicians who have virtually no knowledge of tick-borne disease, because they were "caring and friendly."

Further some want a "local" physician, as if geography is the same as expertise and knowledge.

So how do you pick someone to examine the possibility you have a tick or flea-borne infection?

1) It may take a number of appointments to get better.

2) There is no better use of any income than improving your health and the health of your loved ones.

3) However, are you wasting it on healer after healer who is sincere, but does not have a complete passion to master these illnesses, and a good track record of improving lives, including the lives of very ill patients? I will not debate how

long it takes to kill Bartonella, Babesia and Lyme when they have been missed for twenty years. But it may be that one session will not cure all **your ills.**

The use of herbal treatments without solid follow-up by direct and indirect means needs careful study.

Currently, one finds herbs that are mixed in grain alcohol with a fiftieth of the potency of a capsule, that are supposedly cures to tick-borne disease. In our examination of these inherited treatment failures, we have not found that these low potency alcohol based herbs cure. Others offer high priced herbs and "know" they are successful, and often recommend one size for all adults living on the earth. Often their understanding of advanced herbal processing, standardization and the multiple chemicals in any herb is limited. In any event, in our outcome studies we have found that these herbs at best may limit body infection volume slightly. It is profoundly important to use effective herbs with a tailored, specialized dosage for each individual or you are merely experiencing "mill medicine." If you are self-treating with herbs or if your healer promotes "one-size-fits-all," you are accepting health care inferior to dog medicine.

Advice from web sites and chat rooms usually does not apply to you. No two people are ever to be treated exactly the same.

Most physicians and healers are concerned, and rightly so, when patients seek advice on the Internet. Sometimes you can find mature balanced support from those who are healthy, but not new, advanced and solidly credible information for your medical care. Many leaders in tick infection medicine report they are quoted incorrectly, and that the information is often wrong, sometimes dangerous and wastes time and money.

Practitioners are not aware of current treatment approaches.

Practitioners who follow a year-after-year I.V. treatment approach are not "up-to-date" in their knowledge of Lyme. Ten years of Lyme disease treatment is not acceptable. These so called "cure" treatments often merely lower the body's pathogen load or decrease symptoms without fully eradicating all the different types of infectious agents.

If someone never examines indirect testing for Bartonella, or assumes Bartonella can only make a few skin alterations, they are sadly very dated.

Any proposed treatments that ignore Bartonella means the treatments proposed are not applicable to this decade. It has been very well established that Bartonella is both a highly common vector infection, and is carried in both ticks and many other vectors like fleas. Bartonella is in the ticks that carry Lyme and Babesia.

Further, since we are on the topic of Bartonella, it is stunning to see the immense certainty published in some studies about the complete and perfect effectiveness of azithromycin (Zithromax), rifampin, mycobutin, Levaquin, Cipro, doxycycline or minocycline. When I read these studies I am thankful people are looking to treat this infection that can kill at an unknown frequency, and harm most organs 15-20 ways, but it is a concern that the studies seem to be reasonable, yet the conclusion is simply wrong.

When you read full-time two years, not two months, on this infection, you learn all the new publically defined species, and the new species that infect humans, as well as the immune suppression abilities and realize that brilliant researchers have to understand more about the infections' ability to hide, and suppress each other as well as the limits to test kits before they do a study.

One is reminded of the lovely and compelling studies about Epstein-Barr virus (EBV) as a cause of fatigue and other ills, and how this position as a reported cause of fatigue is simply not true. And any infection or inflammation disorder, in my opinion, can cause EBV to show abnormal results.

So my only point here is to discuss another angle on Bartonella in tick and flea infection troubles.

Routine Bartonella treatments are not effective. So why is the research that shows I was right six years ago ignored?

Right now the infection with more vectors than any infection on earth has one study being done at the National Institutes of Health—it is Bartonella. So we should be stunned if any study is done on the treatments of Bartonella that contradict that Bartonella is very easy to kill? Most clinicians feel Bartonella is trivial and very easy to kill and also easy to remove. I have read these unusually designed and confident papers—often five to ten times.

Let me briefly mention some materials that no one seems to read that undermines the simplistic approaches common in treating Bartonella.

Research shows the common "best treatments" for Bartonella agree with what I published six years ago--they are ineffective. Why? Possibly in part due to Bartonella resistance to the treatment.

The chief mechanisms by which antibiotics work are now found to be undermined by Bartonella. So the treatments published in the past about perfect effectiveness may not have any use now. My study and opinion in 2005 was these were rarely effective in people in 2004.

In new research, antibiotic resistant mutations have been found in *B. henselae, B. quintana and B. bacilliformis*.

In one study 20 new *Bartonella* isolates to fluoroquinolones were examined, and resistance to some quinolones was found. Another author reports: fluoroquinolones alone should not be used for the treatment of bartonellosis since there is an intrinsic low level of resistance due to the gyrA mutation. Moreover, high level of resistance to fluoroquinolones is easily obtained. It is surprising that so many physicians prescribe Levaquin, ciprofloxacin (Cipro) and moxifloxacin (Avelox). These are supposed to have restricted use, including the 4th generation class Avelox. These all have clear tendon damage risks, and a profoundly high risk of C. difficile and MRSA infections. I only see perhaps 1 in 100 patients who are treated with quinolone antibiotics who are also on any probiotic, and only 1 in 500 who are on good probiotics that bind to the wall of the intestines, proliferate and work in synergy.

The facts are that quinolones increase the risk of developing tendonitis and tendon rupture in patients of all ages taking fluoroquinolones. Many quinolones are no longer available due to severe toxicity issues.

Further, azithromycin was effective only until the second passage for *B. henselae* isolates obtained from cats. Other studies show azithromycin, rifampin and quinolone resistance in various Bartonella variants.

Finally, some feel aminoglycosides are the best treatment, but some research tells physicians not to count on an effective use.

Why do guidelines and physicians suggest treatments that may be worthless?

In summary, cat scratch disease does not typically respond well to the cliche options in fair papers. That these troubled treatments are not obvious to very smart MD's, DO's or PhD's shows the terribly poor knowledge they have about Bartonella.

Sample Supporting References

Angelakis E, Biswas S, Taylor C, Raoult D, Rolain JM. Heterogeneity of susceptibility to fluoroquinolones in Bartonella isolates from Australia reveals a natural mutation in gyrA. J Antimicrob Chemother. 2008 Jun;61(6):1252-5. Epub 2008 Mar 10.

Angelakis E, Raoult D, Rolain JM. Molecular characterization of resistance to fluoroquinolones in Bartonella henselae and Bartonella quintana. J Antimicrob Chemother. 2009 Jun;63(6):1288-9. Epub 2009 Apr 15. PMID:19369272

Barbian KD, Minnick MF. A bacteriophage-like particle from Bartonella bacilliformis. Microbiology. 2000 Mar;146 (Pt 3):599-609.

Battisti JM, Smitherman LS, Samuels DS, Minnick MF. Mutations in Bartonella bacilliformis gyrB confer resistance to coumermycin A1. Antimicrob Agents Chemother. 1998 Nov;42(11):2906-13.

Biswas S, Maggi RG, Papich MG, Breitschwerdt EB. Molecular mechanisms of Bartonella henselae resistance to azithromycin, pradofloxacin and enrofloxacin. J Antimicrob Chemother. 2010 Mar;65(3):581-2. Epub 2009 Dec 18.

Biswas S, Raoult D, Rolain JM. Molecular characterization of resistance to macrolides in Bartonella henselae. Antimicrob Agents Chemother. 2006 Sep;50(9):3192–3.

Biswas S, Raoult D, Rolain JM. Molecular mechanisms of resistance to antibiotics in Bartonella bacilliformis. J Antimicrob Chemother. 2007 Jun;59(6):1065-70. Epub 2007 Apr 21.

Biswas S, Raoult D, Rolain JM. A bioinformatic approach to understanding antibiotic resistance in intracellular bacteria through whole genome analysis. Int J Antimicrob Agents. 2008 Sep;32(3):207-20. Epub 2008 Jul 10.

Biswas S, Raoult D, Rolain JM. Molecular mechanism of gentamicin resistance in Bartonella henselae. Clin Microbiol Infect. 2009 Dec;15 Suppl 2:98-9. PMID:20584166

Biswas S, Raoult D, Rolain JM. Molecular characterisation of resistance to rifampin in Bartonella quintana. Clin Microbiol Infect. 2009 Dec;15 Suppl 2:100-1. Epub 2009 Dec 24. PMID:19929979

del Valle LJ, Flores L, Vargas M, García-de-la-Guarda R, Quispe RL, Ibañez ZB, Alvarado D, Ramírez P, Ruiz J. Bartonella bacilliformis, endemic pathogen of the Andean region, is intrinsically resistant to quinolones. Int J Infect Dis. 2010 Jun;14(6):e506-10. Epub 2009 Dec 6.

Meghari S, Rolain JM, Grau GE, Platt E, Barrassi L, Mege JL, Raoult D. Antiangiogenic effect of erythromycin: an in vitro model of Bartonella quintana infection. J Infect Dis. 2006 Feb 1;193(3):380-6. Epub 2005 Dec 27.

Minnick MF, Wilson ZR, Smitherman LS, Samuels DS. gyrA mutations in ciprofloxacin-resistant Bartonella bacilliformis strains obtained in vitro. Antimicrob Agents Chemother. 2003 Jan;47(1):383-6.

Some treatments that cost a good deal of money and time may be ineffective.

For example, the use of hyperbaric oxygen (HBOT) for the treatment of tick-borne infections fails. Results from studies of the use of HBOT in mice are not applicable to humans. To prove that HBOT is useless for the treatment of tick-borne infections, I decided to perform a self-funded study to examine its benefits for the treatment of Lyme (Borrelia), Babesia, Ehrlichia and Bartonella. The family strongly wanted this care but could not afford it, so I paid for them to receive these treatments from David Perlmutter, MD, who believed this would be a successful treatment. After approximately 120 treatments at 2.4 atmospheres for 90 minutes each, administered by very accomplished HBOT techs, the results were not what any expected. Even though the treatments were three times per week at a great facility, the treatment failed.

All participants, after these treatments, still had clear positive findings for all four infections. Therefore, there is no validity to the claim that HBOT "kills" Babesia, Bartonella, Ehrlichia or Lyme disease. I have talked to the late Dr. Fife in detail about his HBOT study and carefully evaluated the HBOT research of Dr. Robert Lombard, who accepted patients on routine antibiotic and antimalarial *treatments while getting HBOT,* which has further confirmed this finding, because people did not return to baseline quickly in four weeks, as expected with double treatment.

I love HBOT treatment for many medical problems, and we know it does kill surgical and some other infections, but it does not cure common tick and flea-borne infections. It may help other aspects of patients' suffering, but I defer that to other physicians and healers.

Many medicines, healing machines and top retail herbal options are of limited help, or are sold at very inflated prices by healers.

Ignoring new data leads to treatment failures.

All medical groups have founders who represent the core beliefs of their organization. These founders are closed-minded about receiving new information. This is simply human nature. For example, different friends who are researchers have performed new surgical techniques or found newer, more useful treatments in many areas of medicine, as have I, and the first response is inertia and a lack of interest. It is so bad, that I discuss new discoveries with patients before physicians.

For example, around 2000, I found a functional "cancer" cure. I found it only because my co-author with a full-time top orthodontry practice asked me firmly to research it along with five other topics. And once I proved it was a solid winner, he shared my paper over and over with oncologists and other cancer experts to get it noticed. If he had not been so driven on this finding, many more would have died from HES or Idiopathic Hypereosinophilia Syndrome. Few exist in the healing professions like my co-author, Dr. Glenn Burkland, who was not only willing to study outside his field, and help find the new serious finding, but also willing to nag people to read and accept this very new information. It is no wonder he is a peerless top clinician and researcher. But we see that excellence often comes from outside clique locations. For example, the only current hospital wing dedicated to tick infection research is at Columbia run by psychiatrist B. Fallon, MD. Indeed, most of those who designed the Infectious Diseases Society of America guidelines on Lyme disease were not infection specialists. They were not afraid to use people with other specialties. Any organization willing to admit that doctors outside their specialization can add information to their guidelines is acting wisely. If neurologists use psychiatrists and psychiatrists use neurologists, in position papers, I feel the papers will be better.

In the same way, I have interests in many specialties, and not mere infection medicine. And yet now I have published eight books on advanced tick-borne infections, all showing new types of information, without an infection fellowship. For some "Lyme-literate" physicians, it took educated patients "throwing a copy" of one of my books at them before they read this new information, and by then **many years had already passed.** Some health care workers believe in a Lyme literate Pope or President, but no such expert exists. Sure, some offer useful information from past investigations. However, no one has mastered modern tick-borne medicine and all the newest co-infection information. And we know from the history of medicine that in every generation that positions from medical "elite" are most often limited and flawed.

Right now I am working on a *Babesia Treatment Update* and a *Three Volume Tick Infections* series, and they are so difficult and involve over 500 pages of references, that I will likely wait until 2013. New data usually comes from those working and reflecting full-time on a topic, and we are quite open to error if we mock such people. I know some have mocked my research and study. I end up treating too many of their patients. I take no delight in saying this alienating statement, but I care more about patients than looking or sounding "professional."

Sick physicians, sick nurses, sick chiropractors or sick herbal physicians (NDs) are trying to treat sick patients.

I have been asked by a number of physicians to share my various impressions of literature reviews of thousands of articles, and they are obviously asking primarily for themselves. They do not want to be patients but want thirty to sixty minute summaries of things that require forty to eight hundred pages to begin to answer.

They are ill themselves and need treatment help. I have asked them to stop treating themselves, and to do an hour consultation with very extensive labs. Most have refused. Tragically, what they could have learned by fixing themselves would have translated into real help for their patients.

My position on these infections fits no one protocol or approach, so I can help any professional regardless of their orientation. In the treatment of tick-borne infections we have limited tools, but enough to offer options other types of healers can accept.

Current treatment recommendations are profoundly flawed or too simplistic.

* I.V. treatments are often used without herbal or synthetic antibiotic cyst busters. Surprisingly, some even mock the notion of spirochete cyst forms.

* The most common treatment for Babesia is 750 mg per teaspoon of Mepron, taken twice a day. This treatment fails in some patients and is too high a starting dose for some people.

* The most commonly used herbal Babesia cures are artemisinin, dihydroartemisinin, or artesunate (for example, Zhang Artemisia from Héprapro.com uses artesunate). The latter involves a "standard" dose of one capsule three times a day. Artemisinin is poor at killing Babesia and three artesunate do not cure most patients. Further, in patients with high systemic inflammation, three artesunate per day may be too uncomfortable. The patient may need some new approaches we have designed to help this very serious problem of chronic high inflammation.

* Azithromycin (Zithromax) is **not** effective at killing Babesia at a mere 500 mg a day. It does kill Babesia at 2,000 mg which was published years ago. All of the approaches listed in infection books and articles can fail at published and recommended doses, even after long trials of treatment.

A lack of two-year blind studies leads to treatment failures for Bartonella. For example, I have found that high doses of Levaquin, rifampin, Zithromax, doxycycline, Mycobutin, acupuncture, Ceftin, Cipro, Avelox, gentamicin, Omnicef, Cumanda and Banderol all fail to cure Bartonella. These antibiotics, along with Rife machines that are used at various optimal frequencies and powers, may lower the body's pathogen load and lead to initial and convincing feelings of improvement, but none of these treatments leads to a cure for Bartonella.

The current tests for Babesia, Bartonella and Ehrlichia are limited.

Some DNA or PCR tests that are processed by a popular East Coast lab often miss a positive infection up to ten times. If a lab needs ten urine or blood samples to show a positive result, it is not functional. Some labs are only fair at tissue PCR testing, when the tissue has clear Lyme, Babesia and Bartonella that can be observed microscopically. This is a diagnostic disaster.

Amazingly, some rely upon large national labs to do manual examinations of red blood cells to look for Babesia and Bartonella. I have never seen a large national lab detect Babesia or Bartonella in over 600 manual smears. No national lab has been able to capture these infections in patients with certain strains of Babesia and Bartonella. I have repeatedly offered to assist them in improving their technology by linking them with hematology experts in tick-borne infections. They did not care that their manual smears were worthless, and I was repeatedly ignored.

The knowledge base about both Bartonella testing and treatment is so poor it borders on the catastrophic.

Bartonella is one of the most common infections in the world. Calling it a "co-infection" may be an error. If anything, Lyme (Borrelia) might be the "co-infection." Bartonella is found in vast numbers of common vectors including dust mites, fleas, flea feces, pet saliva, ticks, etc. Amazingly, it can turn off or lower antibodies to Lyme disease, Babesia, Ehrlichia, Anaplasma and even itself. Bartonella floats in blood and also enters all blood vessel walls without causing a fatal fever, and indeed, actually lowers fevers. It is the ultimate stealth infection. It turns off antibodies, fevers and immune function defense chemicals as it damages organs in anywhere from 15-60 different ways. Many organs can be harmed 15-20 ways and the brain at least 60 ways.

The use of fixed "protocols" or "procedures" in the treatment of tick-borne infections is "machine mill" medicine.

Why? It treats each ill human person as a machine that is built the same and has the exact same problems, which in turn objectifies the patient and flirts with the sociopathic. We see this mindset in serious criminals, who mold people into objects in an effort to fit their skewed perceptions of the world. It is junk medicine to apply a blanket protocol to a unique human body, with a complex and multi-faceted infection cluster and unique biochemical response. Treating in this manner is poor "mill medicine," plain and simple.

Bartonella turns off the production of antibodies to infections like Babesia, Lyme disease and Ehrlichia; it must always be considered in tick and flea medicine.

I would suggest that practitioners learn the 60 different skin patterns that can be created by Bartonella or a mix of Bartonella/Lyme infections. It would also be useful for them to become familiar with the indirect lab markers that are associated with Bartonella infections, as well as those that are associated with mixed Bartonella/Babesia infections, such as IL-6, IL-1B, TNF-alpha, ECP, and VEGF. We discuss clinical patterns that are seen as a result of these lab results in the *Babesia 2009 Update* book and *The Diagnosis and Treatment of Bartonella* book.

Some patients have very few Babesia protozoa parasites, but they are causing serious trouble in their bodies. Practitioners don't recognize them to be a problem, however. Their small numbers cause them to be missed in visual "FISH" exams, PCR and antibody tests. But indirect testing can allow them to be detected.

Most labs don't test for new species of Babesia and Bartonella. Yet there are special ways to detect these infections. Most international labs are unable to test for Babesia duncani or the many other documented species of Babesia (15) or Bartonella (10) that infect humans.

Practitioners cannot rule out the presence of these infection species just because patients test negative for them. One way to reduce treatment failures is to use new medical techniques to detect stealth Babesia. (Babesia can cause symptoms of ongoing fatigue, headaches and weight gain, as well as others, while hindering the treatment of Lyme disease).

The "trick" is simple: a patient is given at least two Babesia killing medications such as Mepron, artesunate or Malarone (given for the proguanil). These medications are used for four days at a dose that both patient and physician feel is worth the risk. Usually, at least one of the medications will kill a few Babesia parasites. Approximately ten to fourteen days later, a follow up lab test is performed, in which blood is drawn and VEGF, TNF-alpha, IL-6, IL-1B, and ECP levels are assayed. ECP is used to kill parasites. The new ECP level is compared to the baseline. If the ECP or TNF-alpha levels rise and VEGF falls, it can be a sign of Babesia "die-off." (Eosinophils release ECP and possibly react to the single-celled parasite Babesia or Babesia debris as if a larger parasite, which is the primary role of Eosinophils—killing large parasites). An increase in either IL-6 or IL-1B is not routine, but an increase after these trials is a sign that suspicions exist for the presence of Babesia.

An added option is to wait six weeks after using this lab technique and have the patient tested for antibodies to Babesia microti or duncani. One juvenile patient with profound illness, who was increasingly disabled after being seen by approximately fifteen physicians, was finally diagnosed in this manner, and after three weeks of triple Babesia treatment, had significant clinical improvement for the first time in six years.

Not being able to detect stealthy, low-volume Babesia is a common problem when treating tick and flea-borne infections. Talented health care workers commonly miss these red blood cell parasites, but this trick usually causes these singled-celled parasites to show up and can save patients from years of failed treatment.

First, look at these five labs below. Alone, they can each be low, normal or high for many reasons. But in tick and flea infection medicine, reading patterns of them can be helpful.

TNF-alpha represents Tumor Necrosis Factor-alpha

IL-6 represents Interleukin 6

IL-1b represents Interleukin 1b

VEGF represents Vasoendothelial Growth Factor

ECP means Eosinophil Cationic Protein

I will not go too deeply into the function of these common labs, except to say that VEGF makes and opens blood vessels. **Bartonella makes VEGF (and so do mold toxins such as those measured reliably by Real Time Labs). If your skin or labs show Bartonella findings and the VEGF is not well above normal, something is likely going on. What could it be? It could be that Babesia is present and suppressing full body blood VEGF levels,** but it does not stop the production in some patients of Bartonella skin markings consistent with the 40 **different** skin markings illustrated in my two-volume color Bartonella book. These markings appear less often in children under nine years old, because they have had less time to develop.

Bartonella suppresses other labs such as the TNF-alpha, IL-6 and IL-1b. So in the presence of only Bartonella and Lyme, these labs are **typically low and often *below* normal.**

Bartonella and Lyme Infection

TNF-alpha	low
IL-6	low
IL-1b	low
VEGF	high

Babesia and Lyme without Bartonella

First, since I believe Bartonella is one of the most common bacterial infections on earth, the notion that Babesia and Lyme would exist without at least one species variant of Bartonella would be unusual. But since Bartonella medicine and lab testing surrounding this powerful stealth infection is 20 years behind the times, the belief that some people have just these two infections is common. So let's discuss what it would look like in this theoretical situation. (This assumes no 15/16-6/5-51 HLA).

TNF-alpha	high
IL-6	normal-high
IL-1b	normal-high
VEGF	low-normal

Babesia and Bartonella Together

TNF-alpha	high

Bartonella lowers the value of this lab, so if it is high, is something driving it high, such as Babesia? It should be low with Bartonella alone.

IL-6	low-normal-high

While Bartonella lowers this, in the presence of Babesia, it may or may not become increased. If it is in the 40th percentile or higher, this is suspicious for Babesia.

IL-1b	low-normal-high

While Bartonella lowers this, in the presence of Babesia, it may or may not become increased. If it is in the 30th percentile or higher, this is suspicious for Babesia.

Please do not assume **both** IL-6 and IL-1b will both go up in the presence of Babesia. **In fact, sometimes only TNF-alpha or IL-6 or IL-1b increases, while the other two remain low.**

VEGF	**low-normal**

Generally even **very low numbers of Babesia will bring high levels of VEGF down.** At times Babesia will reduce VEGF significantly to moderate or low "normal" blood levels in the accepted range of the test.

On occasion Babesia makes VEGF so low it is actually unable to be measured. One new problem with some laboratories is that they have had a new flood of thousands of VEGF tests being done on very ill patients. Some of these have very low VEGF blood levels. So at least one large lab, LabCorp, has revised its normal range markedly downward based on very ill patients. Therefore their new normal range is based on an ill patient population and not healthy and normal patients. The outcome then, if a lab alters the lowest "normal" range to zero, is that they have created a statistical and clinical flaw, much like saying the normal range for human eyes is zero to two. In the same way, some labs actually say a VEGF of **zero** is part of the normal range. Wrong. A VEGF of 31-85 is fine for our purposes here.

The critical point is that Bartonella manufactures VEGF directly or indirectly, creating a *high level of VEGF* in the blood and also in tissues. (Sometimes the skin shows evidence of VEGF). It is the chemical that sometimes causes various red, burgundy and blue blood vessel findings all over the body. If a person has Bartonella alone with Lyme, VEGF is almost always going to be above the normal range. If VEGF is low or normal, one common cause in a person with Lyme disease or ixodes tick exposure risk is a Babesia infection.

Finally, let me merely mention the meaning of ECP or Eosinophil Cationic Protein. It is used by eosinophil cells to kill parasites, but not single-celled parasites as a rule. Sometimes the ECP is in the top 15%. In the presence of effective Babesia killing in about 60 percent of Babesia positive patients, ECP is over the top normal level.

Sample Bartonella Laboratory References

1. Cerimele F, Brown LF, Bravo F, Ihler GM, Kouadio P, Arbiser JL. Infectious angiogenesis: Bartonella bacilliformis infection results in endothelial production of angiopoetin-2 and epidermal production of vascular endothelial growth factor. *Am J Pathol*. 2003;163(4):1321-1327.

2. Dehio C. Recent progress in understanding bartonella-induced vascular proliferation. *Curr Opin Microbiol*. 2003;6(1):61-65.

3. Herremans M, Bakker J, Vermeulen MJ, Schellekens JF, Koopmans MP. Evaluation of an in-house cat scratch disease IgM ELISA to detect bartonella henselae in a routine laboratory setting. *Eur J Clin Microbiol Infect Dis*. 2008. 10.1007/s10096-008-0601-8.

4. Kempf VA, Schairer A, Neumann D, et al. Bartonella henselae inhibits apoptosis in mono mac 6 cells. *Cell Microbiol*. 2005;7(1):91-104. 10.1111/j.1462-5822.2004.00440.x.

5. Lappin MR, Breitschwerdt E, Brewer M, Hawley J, Hegarty B, Radecki S. Prevalence of bartonella species antibodies and bartonella species DNA in the blood of cats with and without fever. *J Feline Med Surg*. 2008. 10.1016/j.jfms.2008.06.005.

6. Mathieu S, Vellin JF, Poujol D, Ristori JM, Soubrier M. Cat scratch disease during etanercept therapy. *Joint Bone Spine*. 2007;74(2):184-186. 10.1016/j.jbspin.2006.05.017.

7. Popa C, Abdollahi-Roodsaz S, Joosten LA, et al. Bartonella quintana lipopolysaccharide is a natural antagonist of toll-like receptor 4. *Infect Immun*. 2007;75(10):4831-4837. 10.1128/IAI.00237-07.

8. Raoult D, Dutour O, Houhamdi L, et al. Evidence for louse-transmitted diseases in soldiers of napoleon's grand army in vilnius. *J Infect Dis*. 2006;193(1):112-120. 10.1086/498534.

9. Resto-Ruiz SI, Schmiederer M, Sweger D, et al. Induction of a potential paracrine angiogenic loop between human THP-1 macrophages and human microvascular endothelial cells during bartonella henselae infection. *Infect Immun*. 2002;70(8):4564-4570.

10. Vermeulen MJ, Diederen BM, Verbakel H, Peeters MF. Low sensitivity of bartonella henselae PCR in serum samples of patients with cat-scratch disease lymphadenitis. *J Med Microbiol*. 2008;57(Pt 8):1049-1050. 10.1099/jmm.0.2008/001024-0.

The Bartonella testing of most national labs is surprisingly poor.

It is stunning to read about so-called "sages" who report that patients don't have Bartonella just because a large lab didn't find antibodies to the infection in their blood.

First, these "sages" do not understand that Bartonella turns off its own antibodies, and that the large labs only check for one (or two) species that infect humans, and their cut-off titers are unrealistically high.

Bartonella FISH testing is now available (except in New York State) from IGeneX and is useful but should never be the only test. Fry Clinical Laboratories has a very sensitive smear that shows Bartonella. We have found that when they report Bartonella, we see indirect labs that are consistent with the presence of Bartonella. These indirect labs are mentioned in a full and complete review of the international PubMed articles on the topic which I have read over many years.

Infections and inflammation decrease insight.

Tick-borne infections routinely destroy patients' ability to have insight into treatments and lead to personality changes and/or rigid resistance to testing. This is largely due to an impaired frontal lobe (the part of the brain involved in self-awareness). Examples of decreased insight are demonstrated by the following situations:

a. Patients feeling like they are cured when they have only experienced partial improvement in their symptoms.

b. Patients intentionally going to practitioners who use inferior labs.

c. Patients refusing, with eccentric resistance, to be tested for tick-borne infections.

d. Patients dismissing positive test results with a wave of their hand.

Some patients insist that their problem is mold alone and not tick-borne infections.

They cannot believe **both** indoor mold and tick-borne infections are important. The idea that one could be causing 80 percent of their symptoms and the other was "the straw that broke the camel's back" is a concept they reject.

Some patients get ill after a flood, large leak or some other water intrusion problem. They feel they are ill only because of mold mycotoxins in their home that have formed 36-48 hours after water intrusion into drywall, insulation, carpeting and other dust or cellulose-filled materials. The EPA reports that 30 percent of US structures have indoor mold. Some of these indoor molds have war-grade chemicals on their surfaces. When the tomb room of the last King of Poland, Casimir IV was opened in Paris in 1973, ten of the twelve scientists who were present died. One survivor had expertise in mold and subsequently found specific toxic mold species. I must confess that as a certified mold investigator and certified mold remediator, I am utterly stunned that many physicians actually dismiss the notion of indoor mold being related to illness.

Here is one example why that is a scientific error.

Mold chemicals from mummies kill tomb researchers

In recent years, some "mold experts" ignoring almost 100% of the 33,000 mycotoxin references in PubMed, and who are also weak on remediation, have received public attention. Others seem to know nothing about the illnesses caused by mold other than 1970's leaky gut issues or spore illness found in severely immune suppressed people who are very rare. We have known for at least 30 years illness can be caused by the chemicals from indoor mold. In medical schools, no one is really taught this information.

Most of us have heard the term "Beware the Mummy's Curse." Many individuals working in archeology or tomb robbery have died soon after opening and entering tombs or handling their contents.

Perhaps the caution began when Lord Carnarvon, an elderly and medically frail expert in Egyptian archeology, was involved in the excavation of King Tut's tomb in 1922. After 5 years, 11 who had entered the tomb were dead.

Since such tombs typically had fruits, vegetables, meats, clothing and furniture, molds would naturally form in these dark places and form spores and their surface toxins that could last thousands of years. The first to enter these tombs, before they were aired out, would get a huge dose of mold toxins.

This seems to be the general belief of scholars from all over the Middle East, Europe and America.

This was further supported by the examination of the mummy of Ramesses II of ancient Egypt, which was examined in a research Museum in Paris in 1976, and over 89 different species of molds were found in or on the mummy. The researchers were fortunately careful enough to be wearing special masks.

One of the most serious recent mold toxin Archeology disasters occurred when the tomb of a famous 15th century Polish leader, King Casimir, was opened in 1973 by 12 researchers. The wooden coffin was heavily rotted inside the tomb. In a few days, four of the 12 were dead. Soon six more died. One of the two survivors was Dr. Smyk who was an expert microbiologist and suffered 5 years with new neurological balance trouble. He studied some tomb artifacts in great detail and found clear Aspergillus and Penicillin species that make dangerous mycotoxins, such as aflatoxins…

Is it any wonder that experts on this topic, like Dr. Barbara Janinka from the Polish Institute of Engineering and Dr.'s Poirier and Feder, in their book *Dangerous Places: Health, Safety, and Archaeology,* remind us of an old observation about archaeology—when you go home after a hard day in the field and blow your nose, you blow out dirt." Feder said, "Clearly you have been breathing it in, and if you have been exposed to molds, spores, or fungi that lay dormant in the earth, there is at least a possibility of being exposed to some nasty stuff."

However, if the reader does not follow the required home, school, office, church or synagogue mold prevention hygiene steps, the same molds that have killed archeologists in the past can become part of your world. And in many cases, in ways much more than a runny nose or red eyes!

Examples of scholars who believe toxic molds like Aspergillus and Penicillium species make poisons like Ochratoxins, and have been responsible for Archeologist deaths include: Dr. Ezzeddin Taha of Cairo University, the Italian physician Dr. Nicola Di Paolo, French physician Dr. Caroline Stenger-Phillip, physician Dr. Hans Merk and microbiologist Dr. G. Kramer—both from Germany.

Sample Supporting References

- news.nationalgeographic.com
- www.quaktestusa.com
- www.catchpenny.org
- B. Janinska. Historical buildings and mould fungi. Not only vaults are menacing with "Tutankhamen's Curse." *Foundations of Civil and Environmental Engineering*. (2002): 43-54. www.unmuseum.org
- meta-religion.com/Archaeology/Africa/Egypt/tut_curse.htm

Residing in a moldy location prevents people from being cured from tick and flea-borne infections.

This significant factor was the catalyst for my decision to co-author two mold remediation books. We have also known since the 1880's that the combination of dust and high humidity leads to mold and bacteria growth indoors. Their presence makes Lyme disease much more difficult to cure.

Only 1 in 1000 physicians has read 500 articles on indoor water intrusion's impact on health. One fascinating article includes possible mold chemicals used in the Vietnam War (Wannamaker, *Military Medicine,* Ch. 24).

Further, we can measure three of the most dangerous mycotoxins in your body. Specifically, in an ELISA test done by Dr. Hooper at his Real Time Laboratory, he routinely finds aflatoxins, ochratoxins and trichothenes in the urine of my mold exposed patients. So for example, the Collier county sheriff building and jail here in Naples is filled with mold, rat urine and rats, and the "remediation" is inept, so many staff are retiring, or going out on disability. No one really cares or has a clue the illness this is causing—they simply are ignorant or do not listen.

This sheriff building and jail had ERMI testing done that was positive. ERMI is a research tool developed by the EPA and the results are serious, but no administrator understands that these employees in Naples, Florida are better when away from the sheriff building because it is apparently a "sick building." So here are the possible causes of illness from our example, the sheriff building and jail of Naples.

A. Mold toxins—there are 33,000 articles on these in PubMed. Anyone who questions the sicknesses caused by mycotoxins is illiterate, a sadistic boss, or an insurance company prostitute. I have seen toxicologists, who have not read a full book or 40 articles on mold water illness, report a sick building is safe. Amusingly, every military field of battle medical book I own has a section on the treatment of mycotoxin poison. The military are not fools.

B. Mold inflammation chemicals—when molds eat, they produce a flurry of substances, and some of these increase inflammation in mammals like humans.

C. Bacteria—water inside any structure is really a disaster. If it is dried very fast, in 36 hours or less, generally no health risks exist. Of course this means in all the locations where the water reached. I was recently an expert in a New Jersey utilities case, and the utilities visitor never realized the water was inside the walls, the kitchen ceiling and around the window structure. Why? Because he could care less. We see the same inept ignorance or sadistic bosses running the Naples Florida jail and sheriff building, which has massive mold found in past inspections and a current EPA designed ERMI test. In the past, visible mold was handled by renovators or "remediators" of which 95 percent in Florida and probably other states are vastly under trained. The jail/sheriff offices also have rat urine which has biologically active water. Over twenty bacteria species create toxins when water is present indoors. For example, you have probably heard that the famous Legionnaires' infections in our treasured veterans were due to water in the hotel's AC ducts. I recall very vividly the outbreak of Legionnaires' in the hotel where I attended meetings monthly. One would think from reading infection books that we know everything about all infections. Such hubris is absurd and quickly dispatched by merely refraining from excess alcoholic beverages.

Indeed, the mortality at the original American Legion convention in 1976 was high despite the closeness of the University of Pennsylvania's elite infectious disease department, who are gifted at telling people they are not ill when they feel ill. Thirty-four died and approximately one hundred-eighty were infected.

Despite the obvious infectious symptoms, the infectious agents were not identified for some time as was the case with HIV. Legionnaires' disease was simply caused by a bacterium that takes advantage of standing water. And it is hardly the only killing bacterium that is present in standing water associated with leaks in a home, school or work structure. Legionnaires' disease is still fatal, but the percentage of people surviving is better in recent outbreaks and single infections. We know that standing water in almost any location has some risk if nothing is present to kill the organisms. So as mentioned, prisons and structures with poor ventilation due to building defects, terribly clogged or cheap filters, or a ventilation system with bends in the ducts, allow for condensation of water in the ducts of the air conditioner system, 'which will allow the infected invisible vapor to infect people very far away, infecting anyone not immune to the strain of bacteria.

Finally, please understand, this is a sample dangerous bacterium associated with still water. It is hardly the only one that can cause illness and death.

D. Bacteria biotoxins—in the section above we focused on the infection of water related bacteria. But these bacteria also make biotoxins. These bacteria toxins are dangerous. One you have heard of is related to food poisoning. It is why some food makes people vomit. However, if a location with these biotoxins is fully dried, the bacteria biotoxins should decay. In contrast, mold biotoxins do not easily decay.

It is a medical error to ignore patients sleeping over 9 hours a day or under 7 hours a day.

Some patients with tick or flea infections need over 9 hours of sleep, or cannot sleep 7 hours. Their complaints of fatigue must be taken very seriously, and one must not assume it is the vague "fibromyalgia" which can also be associated with a wide range of things mentioned in this book.

Papers that accept a Fibromyalgia diagnosis quickly are not advanced 2012 medicine nor do they show full-time study in these areas.

If a patient has significant troubles with fatigue, it is possible the infections or other sicknesses mentioned in this book might apply.

For example, if someone is excessively fatigued, here would be some basic labs to order and the result that might fit with the topics in this book.

- ☐ Low free DHT
- ☐ Low FreeT3
- ☐ High Reverse T3
- ☐ One of the many thyroid system auto-immunity labs
- ☐ ECP is over 2010 top range or unable to be measured
- ☐ Babesia lab that has at least a 5% positive reporting range is indeterminate or positive.
- ☐ Urine Real Time mycotoxins are positive
- ☐ The Western Blot is interpreted in a manner similar to some Chinese physicians—if a band is specific for Lyme, it is Lyme positive.
- ☐ Low free testosterone

- ☐ IL-6 is very low
- ☐ IL-1B is very low
- ☐ Vitamin D is under 39 or very low normal
- ☐ WBC count is under 5.0
- ☐ Platelets are under 190.
- ☐ MSH is in lower 20th percentile. Any range that starts at zero is absurd. Five years ago a zero level was never normal, so the norm was changed due to sick patients. If LabCorp is used, the range of normal is 40-85.
- ☐ VIP is in the low 25th percentile
- ☐ C4a is in excess of normal
- ☐ MMPI is over 300 (a top range of over 300 is an error)

One could add dozens of other tests but these are a start.

If any patient reports that any of these are problems, Babesia, Bartonella and Lyme disease should be considered. But Babesia causes the worst fatigue, and using a massive mill lab to test for Babesia is naive. Patients with positive DNA or PCR testing and visualized Babesia inside cells are usually called negative when their blood is sent to large volume labs.

Lyme has at least one surface biotoxin, the patented BbTox1, and some people cannot detoxify this biotoxin.

Patients with 15/16--6/5--51 HLA patterns and possibly others, are possibly unable to remove Lyme biotoxins (R. Shoemaker) and must take a binder like Cholestyramine, which has been used to bind biotoxins since the 1970's. Other HLA patterns have been identified in 2009 that may be responsible for the body slowly releasing Lyme biotoxins. It is not clear how much of this toxin and other inflammatory chemicals are removed by USP purity clay, activated charcoal, top probiotics, cholestyramine, NAC, Cal-D-Glucarate, Milk Thistle or glutathione.

The research in PubMed over many years shows that one binder will always fail to remove some mycotoxins. So an informed and well-read position is the use of multiple agents.

Many patients who have had tick-borne infections have very high levels of inflammation.

High starting doses of antibiotics exacerbate this problem and complicate healing. Therefore, all starting doses of medications or herbs should be very low and gradually raised to higher levels. Additionally, liver-protecting substances should be given in conjunction with these remedies. Starting at full dosing in a "medically sensitive" patient is akin to committing chemical battery. Reactions to massive die-off of infectious organisms may be confused with allergic reactions and can cause panic attacks, shortness of breath, chest pain and severe migraines. This sloppy, one-size-fits-all approach is common in large practices in which a few major "protocols" are routine.

Medical "Band-Aids" are often required to save a job, a marriage and to care for children, but practitioners don't always prescribe these.

They are often a highly useful component of care, however. Pain, fatigue, severe insomnia, depression and anxiety often increase with die-off reactions or as a result of the presence of the infections. Band-Aid treatments are therefore often useful and helpful for patients. I treat people who run companies, schools, very large families and professional teams. They want to sleep 13 hours per day. They need stimulants for a period of time. The use of natural or synthetic stimulant options is discussed in *The Diagnosis and Treatment of Babesia* (available from Amazon.com or www.LymeBook.com). Patients do not benefit from sleep in excess of 8.5 hours. It may just serve to get them fired!

Health care workers have a huge inability to see the core flaw in all "Lyme," "Babesia" and Human "Bartonella" testing research.

Many physicians are no longer comfortable thinking about tick and flea infections for a wide range of reasons. And if they are very busy, they may only have time to open a book and try what was suggested the year before the book was written. They may also fear using a dose below or above what is listed. Some patients can only handle a lower dose or they get side effects; others do not feel better without a higher dose.

First, I have looked over many sincere and well intentioned studies. The common massive error in these studies is the limited reading and experience that promotes the quasi-religious belief that a lab test can be 100 percent accurate and the researcher can find patients that have pure Babesia, Bartonella, Ehrlichia, or Lyme disease. The reality is that it is absolutely impossible as of 2011 to use simplistic ***direct labs,*** which look for species established by approximately the year 2000 and not after, to determine what infections I just mentioned are present. And we are not even talking about the flood of viruses and other newly discovered different types of infections routinely carried by Ixodes ticks that we know about in 2012 if one is aggressively reading and attending conferences.

Of course some exceptions exist. If a person lives in New York City and has a cat, and never is exposed to anything but concrete and tar, they may just get Bartonella from their pet. And roughly 100 years ago, all southern cattle were destroyed by Babesia, and I believe that was Babesia alone. But these are exceptions.

In summary, studies that ***rule out other infections with the wave of simple PCR or titer lab tests are throwbacks to 1995 medicine.*** Any finding is markedly suspect, first, because tick and flea infections are not spread as mono-infections among humans, and second, since single infections do not exist as a rule, lab results may be skewed by the presence of more than one infectious agent.

Reading and researching the ***indirect labs changed by one or many of these infections*** make it clear you are missing infections if you assume the study population has "a single infection." But this requires years of full-time reading to dent this topic, and not merely a few hours at an infection conference.

Look at some sample ways Bartonella hides and alters immunity to understand how serious it can be to you.

Bartonella can:

- ☐ lower your temperature
- ☐ suppress antibodies
- ☐ make new tissue
- ☐ make new blood vessels or new cavities for blood. This is ***not rare*** if you know how and where to look. Increased VEGF is routine, and if VEGF is not high, one should consider the presence of Babesia immediately.
- ☐ use bacteriophages—small virus outer shells that carry genetic information to defeat host defense mechanisms and allow survival in a host.
- ☐ invade the critically important endothelial cells as targets
- ☐ undermine many cell functions
- ☐ invade cells
- ☐ increase inflammation
- ☐ suppress apoptosis (cell death)
- ☐ stimulate cell reproduction
- ☐ create tumor-like growths
- ☐ impair monocytes so that they no longer devour bacteria properly
- ☐ persistently decrease CD8+ lymphocytes (cancer fighting cells)

- ☐ change adhesion molecule expression (downregulation of L-selectin, VLA-4, and LFA-1)
- ☐ harm some CD8+ T lymphocytes
- ☐ limit antigen presentation in human lymph nodes

This is a highly limited set of examples. Why is this new to people? Why is it unknown to most smart physicians?

Sample Supporting References

Harms A, Dehio C. Intruders below the Radar: Molecular Pathogenesis of Bartonella spp. Clin Microbiol Rev. 2012 Jan;25(1):42-78.

Maggi RG, Breitschwerdt EB. Isolation of bacteriophages from Bartonella vinsonii subsp. berkhoffii and the characterization of Pap31 gene sequences from bacterial and phage DNA. J Mol Microbiol Biotechnol. 2005;9(1):44-51. PMID:16254445

Andersen-Nissen E, Smith KD, Strobe KL, Barrett SL, Cookson BT, Logan SM, Aderem A. Evasion of Toll-like receptor 5 by flagellated bacteria. Proc Natl Acad Sci U S A. 2005 Jun 28;102(26):9247-52. Epub 2005 Jun 13.

Ahsan N, Holman MJ, Riley TR, Abendroth CS, Langhoff EG, Yang HC. Peloisis hepatis due to Bartonella henselae in transplantation: a hemato-hepato-renal syndrome. Transplantation. 1998 Apr 15;65(7):1000-3.

Dehio C. Molecular and cellular basis of bartonella pathogenesis. Annu Rev Microbiol. 2004;58:365-90.

Pappalardo BL, Brown TT, Tompkins M, Breitschwerdt EB. Immunopathology of Bartonella vinsonii (berkhoffii) in experimentally infected dogs. Vet Immunol Immunopathol. 2001 Dec;83(3-4):125-47.

Pulliainen AT, Dehio C. Persistence of Bartonella spp. stealth pathogens: from sub-clinical infections to vasoproliferative tumour formation. FEMS Microbiol Rev. 2012 Jan 9. [Epub ahead of print]

Smith KJ, Skelton HG, Tuur S, Larson PL, Angritt P. Bacillary angiomatosis in an immunocompetent child. Am J Dermatopathol. 1996 Dec;18(6):597-600.

Bartonella has psychiatric and neurology effects in excess of current awareness.

In my TV interview and paper on brain effects, I show Bartonella can cause ADHD, ADD, depression, manic symptoms and severe insomnia.

Here are some other findings summarized. Bartonella can cause:

- ☐ trouble speaking
- ☐ acute neurological disease
- ☐ stroke
- ☐ granulomas or other tissue changes of the brain
- ☐ bacteremia
- ☐ retinitis
- ☐ musculoskeletal disorders
- ☐ liver disease
- ☐ spleen disease
- ☐ muscle myocarditis
- ☐ fever of unknown cause
- ☐ new illness after a blood transfusion
- ☐ Encephalitis lethargica with a possible statue-like, speechless and motionless state. It often creates high fever, sore throat, headache, double vision, delayed physical and mental response, sleep inversion, catatonia and lethargy. In acute cases, patients may enter a coma-like state (akinetic mutism). Patients may also experience abnormal eye movements ("oculogyric crises"), Parkinsonism, upper body weakness,

muscular pains, tremors, neck rigidity, and behavioral changes including psychosis. A vocal tic is sometimes present.

- ☐ Fully normal lymph nodes or enlarged nodes—large nodes are not a routine finding
- ☐ malaise
- ☐ dementia

Sample Supporting References

Becker JL. Vector-borne illnesses and the safety of the blood supply. Curr Hematol Rep. 2003 Nov;2(6):511-7.

Ben-Ami R, Ephros M, Avidor B, Katchman E, Varon M, Leibowitz C, Comaneshter D, Giladi M. Cat-scratch disease in elderly patients. Clin Infect Dis. 2005 Oct 1;41(7):969-74. Epub 2005 Aug 30.

Bloch KC, Glaser C. Diagnostic approaches for patients with suspected encephalitis. Curr Infect Dis Rep. 2007 Jul;9(4):315-22.

Brenneis C, Scherfler C, Engelhardt K, Helbok R, Brössner G, Beer R, Lackner P, Walder G, Pfausler B, Schmutzhard E. Encephalitis lethargica following Bartonella henselae infection. J Neurol. 2007 Apr;254(4):546-7. Epub 2007 Mar 12.

Chan L, Reilly KM, Snyder HS. An unusual presentation of cat scratch encephalitis. J Emerg Med. 1995 Nov-Dec;13(6):769-72.

Centers for Disease Control and Prevention (CDC). Encephalitis associated with cat scratch disease--Broward and Palm Beach Counties, Florida, 1994. MMWR Morb Mortal Wkly Rep. 1994 Dec 16;43(49):909, 915-6.

Cherinet Y, Tomlinson R. Cat scratch disease presenting as acute encephalopathy. Emerg Med J. 2008 Oct;25(10):703-4.

Dreher A, Grevers G. [Cat scratch disease. An overview for the ENT physician].[Article in German]. Laryngorhinootologie. 1996 Jul;75(7):403-7.

Edouard S, Raoult D. [Bartonella henselae, an ubiquitous agent of proteiform zoonotic disease].[Article in French]. Med Mal Infect. 2010 Jun;40(6):319-30. Epub 2009 Dec 29.

Fouch B, Coventry S. A case of fatal disseminated Bartonella henselae infection (cat-scratch disease) with encephalitis. Arch Pathol Lab Med. 2007 Oct;131(10):1591-4.

Genizi J, Kasis I, Schif A, Shahar E. Effect of high-dose methyl-prednisolone on brainstem encephalopathy and basal ganglia impairment complicating cat scratch disease. Brain Dev. 2007 Jul;29(6):377-9. Epub 2006 Dec 15.

Gerber JE, Johnson JE, Scott MA, Madhusudhan KT. Fatal meningitis and encephalitis due to Bartonella henselae bacteria. J Forensic Sci. 2002 May;47(3):640-4.

Glaser CA, Gilliam S, Schnurr D, Forghani B, Honarmand S, Khetsuriani N, Fischer M, Cossen CK, Anderson LJ; California Encephalitis Project, 1998-2000. In search of encephalitis etiologies: diagnostic challenges in the California Encephalitis Project, 1998-2000. Clin Infect Dis. 2003 Mar 15;36(6):731-42. Epub 2003 Mar 3.

Grzeszczuk A, Ziarko S, Kovalchuk O, Stańczak J. Etiology of tick-borne febrile illnesses in adult residents of North-Eastern Poland: report from a prospective clinical study. Int J Med Microbiol. 2006 May;296 Suppl 40:242-9. Epub 2006 Mar 10.

Kusumanto YH, Veenhoven RH, Bokma JA, Schellekens JF. [2 patients with atypical manifestations of cat-scratch disease].[Article in Dutch]. Ned Tijdschr Geneeskd. 1997 Feb 22;141(8):385-7.

Marienfeld CB, Dicapua DB, Sze GK, Goldstein JM. Expressive aphasia as a presentation of encephalitis withBartonella henselae infection in an immunocompetent adult. Yale J Biol Med. 2010 Jun;83(2):67-71.

Marra CM. Neurologic complications of Bartonella henselae infection. Curr Opin Neurol. 1995 Jun;8(3):164-9.

McGrath N, Wallis W. Cat-scratch encephalopathy. Neurology. 1998 Oct;51(4):1239. PMID:9781592

McGrath N, Wallis W, Ellis-Pegler R, Morris AJ, Taylor W. Neuroretinitis and encephalopathy due to Bartonella henselae infection. Aust N Z J Med. 1997 Aug;27(4):454. PMID:9448896

Nishio N, Kubota T, Nakao Y, Hidaka H. Cat scratch disease with encephalopathy in a 9-year-old girl. Pediatr Int. 2008 Dec;50(6):823-4.

[No authors listed]. From the Centers for Disease Control and Prevention. Encephalitis associated with cat scratch disease--Broward and Palm Beach counties, Florida, 1994. JAMA. 1995 Feb 22;273(8):614. PMID:7531250

Noah DL, Bresee JS, Gorensek MJ, Rooney JA, Cresanta JL, Regnery RL, Wong J, del Toro J, Olson JG, Childs JE. Cluster of five children with acute encephalopathy associated with cat-scratch disease in south Florida. Pediatr Infect Dis J. 1995 Oct;14(10):866-9.

Ogura K, Hara Y, Tsukahara H, Maeda M, Tsukahara M, Mayumi M. MR signal changes in a child with cat scratch disease encephalopathy and status epilepticus. Eur Neurol. 2004;51(2):109-10. Epub 2004 Feb 11.

Rombaux P, M'Bilo T, Badr-el-Din A, Theate I, Bigaignon G, Hamoir M. Cervical lymphadenitis and cat scratch disease (CSD): an overlooked disease? Acta Otorhinolaryngol Belg. 2000;54(4):491-6.

Singhal AB, Newstein MC, Budzik R, Cha JH, Rordorf G, Buonanno FS, Panzara MA. Diffusion-weighted magnetic resonance imaging abnormalities in Bartonella encephalopathy. J Neuroimaging. 2003 Jan;13(1):79-82.

Skarphédinsson S, Jensen PM, Kristiansen K. Survey of tickborne infections in Denmark. Emerg Infect Dis. 2005 Jul;11(7):1055-61.

Tattevin P, Lellouche F, Bruneel F, Régnier B, De Broucker T. [Bartonella henselae meningoencephalitis].[Article in French]. Rev Neurol (Paris). 2001 Jul;157(6-7):698-700.

Trelles JO, Palomino L, Trelles L. [Neurologic form of Carrion's disease. Clinical-anatomical study of 9 cases].[Article in Spanish]. Rev Neuropsiquiatr. 1969 Dec;32(4):245-306. PMID:5384732

Weston KD, Tran T, Kimmel KN, Maria BL. Possible role of high-dose corticosteroids in the treatment of cat-scratch disease encephalopathy. J Child Neurol. 2001 Oct;16(10):762-3.

Tick and flea infection medicine is not simple if you study each infection in ticks and fleas thoroughly.

Let me share my bias since, unlike some who had no training in the foundations of their thinking due to their overloaded science trainings, I have some sense of my biases. The first is I do not see tick and flea infection medicine as being as simplc as a cold or a strep throat. I see it like HIV, a very large non-fatal third degree burn, or a massive car accident.

First, in keeping with one of my beloved Master's professors Harvie Conn at Westminster, who taught me Kuhn's *The Structure of Scientific Revolutions,* I used hyperbole to allow you to hear me. HIV is worse than tick infections, even if you have not been treated for your insect bite in thirty years. But you get the larger point that these complexes of injected infectious agents are not as simple as a strep throat.

With each passing year of full-time reading, I feel that this is a super-specialization. So a course, a week of lectures, or following an infection specialist on rounds for two weeks is not training, it is merely learning some basic ideas. But my appeal is the tick infection complex of infections is not basic.

This is a problem. If health care practitioners haven't spent 3,000 hours learning about this complex, emerging area of medicine, one that requires a great deal of study in years, then their patients need to find practitioners that are serious about it, instead of someone who is just "doing them a favor" by simply running a few tests.

If I had HIV, I would fly into Washington DC to see a top expert in this infection. I would not want someone who is "somewhat interested" in this disease.

Some patients relapse due to "treatment fatigue," meaning, they are taking too many pills each day even if some are just supplements.

I respect those that try to offer hope and encourage people by telling them that all tick and flea infections are easy to cure. But I also respect those that keep treating in one of many ways when the patient is not back to normal. However, this latter group is often on so many supplements that the patient feels exhausted from simply swallowing all the pills.

I have treated people who have seen all types of doctors with an interest in these infections. Some treated them for a month and others treated them longer.

My appeal to all healers is that asking someone to take 30 pills a day for longer than 2 months is a turn off, so be sure they really need it *or they will get fed up*. For example, some very ill patients may be on I.V. antibiotics or I.V. nutrients for an extended time, and any improvement clinically appears to be over, but some keep treating—I.V.

Others have various healers such as NDs, Chiropractors and integrative physicians, who feel that various supplements can be of use, and have Ms. Levin and Mr. Donaldson taking 40 pills per day. Others waste money on testing that we already know. For example, when I did a toxic water study, I realized every one of my patients had at least three metals above the "healthy" range. So I stopped testing for heavy metals after this was found in about eighty people—they are in all our bodies, and no test is needed to show what is true of all in industrialized nations.

So just give them what prevents clots, strokes, heart attacks, and cancer and lowers inflammation and also give them something for depression, agitation, panic, insomnia, and focus defects. It is a serious problem if they lose their job due to an inability to function.

Many natural and synthetic stimulants are available and should be discussed with your physicians or other health care workers.

So only give what is needed and what the labs show is low in terms of nutrients and hormones so as to keep people from getting fed up and putting them at the end of their treatment rope. This is what happens when practitioners do not treat them fully and effectively at the beginning of their treatment. They get treatment fatigue. Patients should consider a short treatment break, and discuss this option frankly with their health care providers. They should not confuse cure with improvement.

If you are opting for short tick infection care, this is not an issue. However, we all know some patients feel your standard approach helped partly, and want to continue care. It is your presuppositions and your bias for finding truth that will determine what you do. And I will defend you whatever you decide.

The treatment dose that "stuns organisms" is not the same dose that leads to a cure.

Sandy read a book on Babesia I wrote, and could not get anyone to give her a trial of an anti-malarial drug. So because she felt her signs and symptoms fit Babesia [See my Bartonella, Babesia and Lyme disease checklist book on Amazon.com], she purchased some artesunate and tried it herself. It was a modest dose, but ***far too high as a starting dose*** based on my Chinese connections and my own Artemesia and artesunate book research.

Sandy had new severe fatigue, a new severe headache, and chills and sweats. She strongly felt this was consistent with an effective dose, and a top Chinese MD agreed with her. In two days, all her symptoms were gone, and she "felt the best" in her life. She then stopped her herbal malaria medication.

One way to understand Sandy's report is to understand what she did. She took an herbal Chinese drug called "sweet wormwood" [it is **not** wormwood] and she had many symptoms that were new and these started 90 minutes after her artesunate self-trial—a semi-synthetic derivative of the Artemesia grown all over the world, such as in Wisconsin for our troops. And so I believe she felt poorly not from the medication, but from its ability to kill a protozoa or a single-celled parasite like Babesia. But why would she feel so much better and feel ill for a full 48 hours after taking the artesunate?

I believe the reason is simple.

A cure is not a mere reduction in bacterial load or stunning the infection. For example, using Bicillin LA 1.2 million units once a week, without a cyst buster may make someone feel better, but are you sure Lyme cysts do not exist? Are you willing to bet your family's health that it is unlike syphilis which has clear cysts? My bias is frank and open: cysts seem very likely from a review of other spirochetes and some Lyme disease research. And this has not been an area of primary research, so dismissing the idea seems confusing. So my appeal is the possibility of leaving some "Lyme seeds" might be unwise. And people may relapse not merely due to repeat infections, or inflammation residue, but due to active cysts.

It you are leaving cysts you will probably not fully cure patients of Lyme disease. So months or years after receiving "appropriate treatment," the levels of the body's cancer-fighting cells, marked by some as the CD 8/57, may still be under 90. Further, Vitamin D levels can fall into the lower 15th percentile due to active infection and cause an increase in cancer risk and thinning bones. These latter two indirect tests might be associated with Lyme disease and possibly other tick-borne infections. (The C4a test is definitely **not** specific for Lyme, since the presence of many infections or inflammation increases it, but it should probably not be in the top 95 percent or never above normal range).

Cynical relatives, friends or other health care workers defame some healing experts who are actually helping the patient.

You are getting better, or you relate to a physician, but others use the following types of put downs.

The doctor costs too much according to some relatives or strangers. I have insurance—the best in my state. And non-surgeons have never spent over 20 minutes with me, including "intakes" in many years. The real use of my insurance has been paying for covered very expensive surgeries and hospital costs.

Perhaps in your experience you had other healers who took your insurance. But too often I hear that the physicians seem to have "no real interest" in your problems and "did not help or listen fully," or simply passed you on to a "nice" physician extender such as a physician assistant or a nurse.

Having someone listen is very serious. Having a sub-specialist physician listen for over 30 minutes is very rare. They might not be the smartest and may not figure out all your troubles, but being heard matters. I am ashamed to say, at times, I feel I "know what people are thinking," and respond too fast, and it turns out I did not hear them accurately. It really takes time to hear a patient fully.

Others in your life or total strangers insult the healer because you are not getting better. It is true many healers do not know what they are doing, or do not know more than how to do simple screening. But sometimes your family and friends forget you were sick a very long time when you came for care. And extensive labs--not just a few tubes of blood--showed you had multi-body system defects. So if someone is disabled, I do not see anyone from any camp, group or tradition raising the functionally dead patient in a wheelchair in a single season. Any physician who is even willing to try to help someone who is a possible walking malpractice case should get a parade, because if the person continues to do poorly, you often see two undertakers—one for the ill patient and one for the attacked

MD. It is one reason my Canadian patients tell me the sick are often rejected as patients during intakes by family physicians.

Self-treatment rarely leads to your cure.

We all know you should not be your own lawyer. And medicine is 500 times more complex than one state's law. Being a top physician is not merely about the physician's cognitive abilities, but it is about the broadness of that physician's academic research in medicine and medical biochemistry. Due to the explosion of information about tick-borne diseases, I read 50 hours a week, and feel I am falling behind.

Some reject "experts" due to cost even when they use physician extenders--their level of expertise is much less. Others search the land of all answers--the Internet. But the Internet also has every answer, including utter nonsense. And no group has the corner on false medicine. It is so easy to say this ultra-conservative group with only 100 percent synthetic drug options is the right thinkers, but you would be markedly wrong. Others feel only "rebels" offer effective treatment options, but their proof is "Ms. Jones felt better on treatment F."

So if you are going to treat yourself, who will play the pipe to lead you? Some health care practitioners seem too narrow in their approach to treatment, while others are open to virtually everything. So patients get into a medical boat and push themselves out to sea. They read like crazy. They try treatments A through T. They read testimonials of hundreds of patients. They try a wide range of non-prescription options. Some days, weeks or months, they feel better. Other weeks, they don't feel so good. They are upset. They ask themselves, "Why do I have to do all the work and learning?" This is not a good place for them to be. People exist who have already explored 98 percent of the things that those with Lyme are going to explore over the next ten years. They need mentors.

In many of my books and many Internet sites, patients can read about preventing flea and tick bites.

I believe it was Nadelman who proposed that longer term illness was the result of repeated bites. He is quite correct in pointing out that repeated bites happen far too much.

Robert is a hunter. Susan is a hiker. They both love the outdoors passionately. Both were diagnosed with a tick or flea infection of some type. They were given treatment. And they went back to the outdoor living they love. But they only changed their behavior a little bit.

If they use protection it is "spotty."

a. Both own a dog, but neither makes sure the tick and flea killing protection is up to date. They may miss the application date by 2 or 3 weeks at times. When asked, they blame the "busyness" of life.

b. Both are fine having their dog in their bedroom, and when asked to be "honest," both admit to "occasionally" allowing the dog into the foot of the bed and allowing the dog to "kiss" their face or fingers with saliva.

c. Robert reports using permethrin on his hunting clothes last season. He has washed these clothes, but has no idea the permethrin potency he applied to his hunting clothes, and does not know how many times they have been washed. So he has no idea if a tick can crawl onto his skin or if the clothing will kill it in a second.

d. Susan does apply permethrin to her "running shoes and socks" but does **not** realize it must be fully dry to work. She also does **not apply any type of protection above her ankles** due to fear of "cancer causing chemicals."

e. Neither looks over their dogs for fleas or ticks for more than 45 seconds after time outside.

f. Neither looks over their body other than a quick look at their naked body just before getting into the shower or the bathtub. When asked if they "inspected" their body after walking, running or hunting, they actually both smiled. The concept seemed amusing.

g. Both have used DEET but primarily for mosquito contact and "occasionally" to prevent tick bites.

h. Both really did not understand the simple basics about permethrin. For example, permethrin is an insecticide derived from the chrysanthemum family of plants. You do not put it on your skin, but apply it to clothing and allow it to dry before use—skin chemicals denature it so skin contact is not advised. It will not "spook" animals for viewing pleasure or during hunting, since it is odorless. It can survive washing, but the number of washings allowed is related to the concentration. It can stun or kill ticks based on the percentage on clothing and contact duration. Some feel it may have side effects, such as those experienced by those who used it in the Gulf War, but these soldiers were exposed to many other things as well.

i. Susan has used an herbal mix of cedar, geranium, cilantro and another essential oil. She was unsure if it was of any use. What would you say to her? It matters because if you do not understand prevention of tick, flea or insect bites, depending on the location, she could become very ill.

Therefore let me propose some tentative thoughts from the research. I do not claim it is perfect or complete.

First, many feel we need to look at mosquito and tick products differently, meaning, a substance that repels a mosquito may not repel a tick. I hope this is obvious. Many well intentioned people confuse these very different insects. Simply, it is much harder to repel ticks.

Second, we have some research that suggests some organic substances and new substances are as good as DEET or better.

Here are just a few summary findings:

a. The oil of J. communis was nearly as potent as DEET according to top researcher John Carroll writing in 2011 (J Vector Ecol. 2011 Dec;36(2):258-68).

b. Many authors and studies report that DEET needs very high potency to have any meaningful repelling effects against ticks—at dosing far above what is effective against mosquitoes. Some suggest, for example, that high concentrations at 35% may not work to repel ticks, at least not after an hour, and also complain that it melts synthetic clothing, packaging and may have health risks.

c. Semmler reports in Parasitology Research (2011) that saltidin, p-menthan-diol and IR 3535 showed long-lasting effects, and the combination of saltidin and Vitex extracts was very good. [Saltidin is icaridin which is also called, "picaridine or KBR 3023" and is also sold as "Bayrepel." Vitex is an herb with many names, many proposed uses over many centuries and a full discussion would be tangential].

d. Zhang and Klun report that Isolongifolenone is easily synthesized from inexpensive turpentine oil and is cheaper and safer, and is at least as effective as DEET. If this were true, a higher concentration might be worth researching. (2009)

e. Dr. Bissinger published that the EPA approved an extract from wild tomatoes, 2-undecanone, now called, "BioUD," which is 200 to 400 percent more powerful at repelling ticks than DEET (*Exp Appl Acarol*. 2009).

In summary, many herbal derivatives, particularly in the oil or liquid forms which "off-gas" as their means of repelling ticks, include these sample substances mentioned above. The most pronounced effects were observed for the oils of citronella, cloves and lily of the valley. These three at specific concentrations or doses were reported as repelling ticks as effectively as DEET. Further, these substances are not single oils, and some parts were significantly more effective at repelling. For example, parts of citronellol, geraniol (oil of citronella and lily of the valley) and eugenol (oil of cloves) showed pronounced repelling effects along with phenethyl alcohol which is found in small amounts in the oil from lily of the valley. This was reported by Swedish professors, Thorsell, Mikiver and Tunon in 2006 in *Phytomedicine*.

What these three Swedish researchers report reflects a thread in other papers, specifically, if essential oils or other types of oils that can become vapors to make contact with ticks, and are effective at repelling or killing ticks, they can replace DEET. Using these oils, either alone or in combinations, and perhaps with higher dosing, individuals can successfully repel ticks from their skin with greater safety than DEET.

In conclusion, some individuals who are infected with Bartonella, Lyme, Babesia or any other tick infections become fair at protecting themselves. Learning how to prevent repeated bites merely takes thirty minutes of Internet study. It is worth the time. But the first lesson is realizing that the most common infectious tick is very small and requires close attention—not merely a ten second glance as you rush into the shower or bathtub.

Here is a sample case of how sometimes a tick infection cluster is highly complex in body effects.

Thomas Nolan is an FBI worker. He has been struggling with some fatigue, headaches and fair quality sleep for six months.

He has seen about two dozen physicians.

He has some red papules and skin tags on his physical. Further, he is unable to do a heel to toe walking test or one leg raise test well enough to pass a field sobriety test. So if a sheriff or police officer with a High School education did a medical exam on him to determine if he was on drugs or alcohol, he would fail and go to jail. He also has some very slight nystagmus or horizontal jerking of the eye that is borderline positive, which could also result in a DUI arrest. He does not drink or use illegal drugs.

Mr. Nolan's labs showed:

- ☐ a WBC of 4.6 – a low normal
- ☐ A free testosterone abnormally low
- ☐ A DHT or dihydrotestosterone level abnormally low
- ☐ Anticardiolipin is positive
- ☐ ANA is high normal
- ☐ DHEA is within the normal range but very low
- ☐ VIP is undetectable
- ☐ C4a is 5780 or above normal
- ☐ Vitamin D level of 28 or low
- ☐ CD 57/8 is in the low normal range
- ☐ TNF alpha is 1.4

- ☐ IL-6 is in lower 10% or normal range
- ☐ IL-1B is unmeasurable
- ☐ ECP is borderline high
- ☐ VEGF is 120
- ☐ Lyme ELISA is negative
- ☐ Lyme Western blot is "negative" with a positive 31 and 39 band
- ☐ Antibody testing for Bartonella, Babesia, Anaplasma is negative
- ☐ Ehrlichia titer is positive in one test
- ☐ MMP-9 of 437 which is too high, but called normal in the reference range
- ☐ EBV positive
- ☐ C-peptide high
- ☐ C-reactive protein high
- ☐ HLA DR/DQ of 16-5 and 4-3 according to QUEST laboratory. (Quest requires two codes for all five HLA results. These results are identical to LabCorp results)
- ☐ CMV positive
- ☐ HHP-6 positive

I am not going to tell you some of the many possible reasons for these results. It is likely fair to say that it is rare to find a physician who understands the meaning or possible meanings of this information from Mr. Nolan. Anyone who mocks them by saying they are "nonsense" and that each of these labs has "many possible reasons" is half correct. None are nonsense but **each has many possible causes.** However, such comments reveal an inability to see meta-patterns in patients who are not getting better. My only point here is to show in a simple example that systemic infections over time have very dynamic effects, and that tick and flea infections might be a super specialization in medicine. If some of these labs and issues are foreign, it may be a sign of a very complex biochemical domino effect of tick and flea infections that is not appreciated by busy clinicians only trying to keep up with insurance codes and a 50-hour per week full-time practice.

The creative ways to decrease the numbers of Ixodes ticks and to decrease infections in humans from them are markedly flawed.

An important book of medicine in 2011 was R. Ostfeld's *Lyme Disease: The Ecology of a Complex System*. In this book he mentions many strong insights for Lyme disease prevention that includes comments that Lyme diagnosis, prevention and treatment is primitive in each area, and is unimpressed with treatments that are fifty years old. He considers the knowledge of Babesia transmission very primitive without even a good list of reservior hosts. Frankly, he feels the ecological science surrounding Ixodes ticks and Lyme is filled with blind faith convictions which rejected superior science over past decades and made Lyme disease a deer and mouse disease, which is false.

He reminds us that part of the cause of the Black Death or Plague was close proximity of fleas and rats to humans, and the increase of defragmented forests and brush which increases contact between humans and ticks and lowers species diversity, with the immense loss of predators like wolves and cougars who would remove large numbers of tick-carrying small mammals. Effective carriers of infected ticks like chipmunks, shrews and rodents thrive in fragmented locations such as homes and schools with small strips of woods or brush near structures with people. Birds which can carry Ixodes ticks effectively are also more common in fragmented areas with construction and wild brush being mixed in small areas.

Ostfeld strongly opposes the idea of deer being at the center of tick infections, and mentions that research exists in which ***over 70 percent of the deer are removed from islands so the deer cannot be replaced easily as on the mainland, and the infectious rodents actually carried more ticks. Deer removal solutions, such as expensive deer fences or aggressive hunting,*** give very "inconsistent" results, and initially may increase infections. The notion of Lyme and other diseases as "deer infections" is wrong and too simplistic. It is also false that white footed mice are critical for transmission of tick infections. They are immensely easy to catch and due to hairless ears the ticks are vividly clear to researchers. Ostfeld expresses, repeatedly, that faith-like "science" claims regarding carriers and ticks were false. For example, according to various beliefs about North-East USA coastal limits, weather and optimal tick locations it was initially felt that the cold Midwest and Texas and California would **not** be states with high number of infections, yet they are states with many infectious Ixodes ticks.

Solutions to decrease infections, such as 4 pillar posts with tick killers next to "deer" food are not merely "deer devices," because many animals eat from them. Also cotton ball devices with miscellaneous insecticides to kill ticks in rodent nests fail according to high quality studies (Daniels 1991, Stafford 1992). Further, these products along with "bait boxes" are used by many other mammals and not merely mice. My impression of Ostfeld is that he supports an "all of the above" approach, with a full rejection of any notion that this is a deer and white footed mouse disease as immensely simplistic and refuted. He seems troubled by the time wasted by the focus on these two core animals.

Some animals are useful at lowering Ixodes ticks such as opossums, who can eat 5,300 larval ticks a week (pg 127), and some types of birds which kill ticks based on their grooming. Gray squirrels are also poor vectors for tick infection in humans. But he is not suggesting we drop thousands of opossums as a tick control solution.

He reports that burning of wild areas is not effective at reducing infections from ticks.

Using Guinea hens as an approach to reducing tick infections is not an informed option since they only eat adult Ixodes ticks in thin growth areas like lawns--younger forms such as nymphal forms are not reduced in lawns that have these hens compared to lawns without them. Adult Ixodes ticks are not the primary cause of human infections. The use of a Nematode parasite is also an approach recommended to reduce Ixodes ticks, since Ostfeld reports they are also only effective against adult ticks.

He reports that while predators may play a role in control, rodent food profoundly promotes Ixodes tick population growth. So for example, acorns on the forest floor may matter more than raptors like owls and hawks. Some trees may be less supportive of rodents such as birches and most conifers which have seeds too small for rodent food.

Vaccines against tick bites include the same chemicals that make tick bites painless and invisible. He proposes vaccines against tick antihistamines, anti-coagulants, pain killing chemicals and anti-inflammatory chemicals in tick saliva.

While some focus on deer control approaches, at times the number of acorns eaten by mice was a better predictor of Lyme disease than deer numbers.

Ostfeld does feel that having diversity in every aspect of forests may be helpful in some locations. He believes that having many animal varieties likely decreases infection rates rather than having the limited varieties of animals and birds that can survive in small, fragmented green areas between homes or other structures. Further, many ticks escape being killed by some proposed tick control approaches by living deeper in the floor of a wild vegetation area. Ostfeld also suggests that the fungal species Metarhizium anisopliae and Beauveria bassiana can kill ticks and may offer promise. (pp. 179-80).

Organic Tick "Pesticides" and Oils

MAY 2012 ADDENDUM:

Here are some new options for yard and area spraying:

The **F52 strain** of the Metarhizium anisopliae fungus was mentioned above but without a strain. It may matter what strain is used, which occurs naturally in soil.

Nootkatone is an essential oil from Alaskan Yellow Cedar and is effective at killing infectious ticks.

Grapefruit derivatives are also very toxic to ticks.

Cedar oil is not really available for large lawn use since it only exists in cosmetic purity and is expensive. No cedar oil is made at high volume use for lawns that is cost effective.

A garlic spray does suppress tick activity for around two weeks.

A rosemary oil product, called EcoEXEMPT, will eradicate ticks for at least two weeks.

DR. SCHALLER DOES NOT SUPPORT OR OPPOSE THESE OPTIONS.

On the Internet see: scientists-find-fungus-that-kills-lyme-disease-carrying-ticks.

Tick and flea-borne infections cause isolation.

They ruin relationships due to the sick person's fogginess, poor insight, depression, various addictions, rage, anxiety, extreme hostility, or because the individual refuses to get treatment. These infections can even sometimes provoke violence in those infected. This hinders recovery.

I believe Bartonella is likely the worst cause of these problems, but Lyme and Babesia and the die-off reactions that they cause can also increase them.

Isolation leads to decreased treatment options because wisdom and financial support often comes from communities. A mobile society, such as is found in the USA as compared to the Czech Republic, can decrease supports for solid medical wisdom and financial options.

Slow physical decay and the slow alteration of a personality can ultimately lead to unemployment, jail for impulsive actions, divorce and the loss of family relationships and friendships. This, in turn, leads to profound isolation in sickness. Isolated humans, as Mother Teresa often said, are the poorest beings on earth.

Checklists for Bartonella, Babesia and Lyme Disease

All of these checklists are based on over a thousand articles for each infection. Therefore, these are not academically loose lists. Many smart and talented clinicians are unable to diagnosis these infections indirectly, so signs and symptoms for one tick or flea-borne infection will be reported as another infection.

No human on earth at this time could do a **perfect** checklist for these three common infections. But it is hoped researchers and research clinicians will improve on this effort in the coming decades.

The Bartonella Checklist

Increasing Suspicion of an Emerging Stealth Infection

James L. Schaller, M.D., M.A.R.

Introduction

In 2011 a new human Bartonella species was added to the over thirty-five Bartonella species currently publically published in Genetic Data banks. It was discovered and highlighted by the talented veterinarian researcher Edward Breitschwerdt. He has said things more clearly than the ideas I was pondering in 2005, while doing most of the research for my Bartonella book. He said simply, but with devastating and highly useful clarity, that **Bartonella testing is terrible, the treatments are poor,** it is typically found on the outside of red blood cells, and the current research on Bartonella is pathetic—one study at NIH. If this was not enough, he said in 2011, **"Bartonella is carried by more vectors than any infection on the earth."** So it is hardly a backdoor "co-infection." Perhaps Lyme is the "co-infection."

Recently, the German researchers Kaiser and Riess summarized Bartonella research in this manner: after 2 decades of Bartonella research, knowledge on transmission and pathology of these bacteria is still limited. Bartonella species have emerged to be important pathogens in human and veterinary medicine.

Why create a checklist when a physician can just order an antibody test? First, I have found at times, Bartonella can turn off its own antibodies, and those caused by other tick and flea-borne infections in humans. In a study of sixty-one Bartonella infected dogs, Perez and Maggi reported recently that most Bartonella infected dogs **did not have detectable Bartonella antibodies.**

The criteria listed below may have causes unrelated to Bartonella. For example, each year more studies show the presence of poly infections, and this raises the problem of which infection is causing what symptom, sign or lab test change. For example, most tick infections can cause headache or fatigue. Knowing which infection is the cause does become clear if you are doing very advanced treatments that are designed to kill only one infection. The limitation of these poly infection studies is that typically the testing detection rate for each tick or flea-borne infection is not over 95% for all possible species and strains possibly infecting humans.

However, since Bartonella can disable and kill healthy people, the **checklist below is set to catch virtually every infected patient.** This is neither right nor wrong. Philosophy, sociology, presuppositions, medical fashion and psychology usually all play a role in setting cut offs for a diagnosis. All science is guided by presuppositions, and that is why even math research is guided by a wide range of variables. **In medicine, psychology, philosophical assumptions and sociology control all of medicine** but are unappreciated due to a lack of training. **See Kuhn's *The Structure of Scientific Revolutions* exceptionally summarized at the following link: http://des.emory.edu/mfp/Kuhn.html**

THE BARTONELLA CHECKLIST

James Schaller, M.D., M.A.R.

(Please Check Any Symptoms That Apply)

PSYCHIATRIC AND NEUROLOGICAL

- ☐ Current anxiety that was not present at age ten
- ☐ Current depression not present at age sixteen
- ☐ Knee-jerk emotional responses worse than past decades and worsening
- ☐ Brain fog
- ☐ Depression
- ☐ Depression that is not **fully** controlled on **routine anti-depressant doses,** or high dose antidepressants are required to control mood [**Improvement of mood** or being "less depressed" is not successful depression treatment.]
- ☐ Anxiety is poorly controlled with average dosing
- ☐ Depression is poorly controlled by reasonable treatment trials.
- ☐ Suicidal feelings or routine thoughts of death
- ☐ Crying
- ☐ Obsessive thoughts or fear in excess of event
- ☐ Obsessive thoughts that intrude into the mind which are in excess of normal
- ☐ A decrease in pleasure
- ☐ Rage worse with time
- ☐ Irritability worse with time

- ☐ Impatience is greater when compared to ten years ago [in a child--any irritability in excess of what is common for most children with an identical age].
- ☐ Cursing or hostile speech that is worse over time
- ☐ Increased addictions that are very resistant to typical recovery ranges
- ☐ Increased impulsivity in contrast to past years or past decades
- ☐ Severe neurological disorders without a clear cause
- ☐ Severe psychiatric troubles that do not seem to fit with the diagnostic criteria or there is trouble controlling symptoms with treatment
- ☐ New physical, emotional or verbal abuse in the home which was not present in the past
- ☐ Panic attacks that were not present at ten years of age
- ☐ Anxiety medication has to be increased to **very high levels** to continue past benefit
- ☐ Diagnosed as having bipolar disorder, but do not fit the criteria well
- ☐ Any psychiatric disorder that also shows **medical pathology in laboratory tests**
- ☐ Restlessness
- ☐ Combative behavior
- ☐ A parent, grandparent, child or sibling with suicide attempts
- ☐ A parent, grandparent, child or sibling who has started physical or extreme verbal fights
- ☐ Intermittent confusion

- ☐ Seizures
- ☐ Brain lesions seen on a brain scan such as an MRI or CT of the head
- ☐ Short term memory deficits
- ☐ Difficulty in learning new information

DERMATOLOGY OR SKIN

- ☐ Persistent rashes that last over 3 weeks
- ☐ Nodules under the skin
- ☐ Hyper-pigmentation or dark areas of skin which were not present at birth
- ☐ Hypo-pigmentation or obvious light areas of skin
- ☐ Unexplained hair loss
- ☐ Spontaneous breaks or holes in the skin as small as a millimeter
- ☐ Skin ulcerations
- ☐ Stretch marks in eccentric locations, e.g., arms, upper side under armpit, around armpit or on the back
- ☐ Stretch marks filled with red, pink, purple or dark blue color which are not caused by pregnancy or weight loss [remember, many with many pregnancies or weight loss do not have 20 stretch marks]
- ☐ Any skin markings or growths **greater** than most people
- ☐ Blood vessels or color on skin **greater** than most people
- ☐ Red papules of **any** size

- ☐ Skin tags including ones removed by a dermatologist or shaved off
- ☐ Unusual blood vessels of any kind including inside organs such as bladder or intestinal walls
- ☐ Any skin finding in excess of 95% of most humans
- ☐ Skin findings showing increased blood vessels of any size
- ☐ Skin findings showing increased tissue formation that is increased over the flatness of surface skin [This may be due to Bartonella, untreated Lyme disease, or both infections and systemic inflammation]
- ☐ Skin showing blood vessels that are too large or too many for **the location of the blood vessels**, e.g., surface thigh and calf skin with very thick surface blood vessels or legs, upper arms or shoulders have explosions of many fine blood vessels
- ☐ Burning skin sensations [this may have many causes].
- ☐ Itching without a clear cause and which is hard to control and remove
- ☐ Skin erosion without a clear cause such as a fire, fall or chemical burn
- ☐ Minor cuts or scratches which heal slowly
- ☐ Very slow healing after a surgery
- ☐ “Granulomas” or balls of tissue
- ☐ Formication or feelings of being bitten by bugs or bug sensations on skin with no bugs on the skin

EYE

- ☐ Retina infection
- ☐ Retina infarct or dead tissue in the back of the eye
- ☐ Neuroretinitis or inflammation of the retina and optic nerve in the back of the eye
- ☐ Uveitis or inflammation of the middle layer of the eye or the interior eye
- ☐ Papilledema or swelling of the optic nerve as it enters the back of the eye due to raised intracranial pressure
- ☐ Stellate maculopathy
- ☐ Acute blurred vision
- ☐ Sudden and/or significant change in vision

HEART

- ☐ Endocarditis or inflammation of the heart
- ☐ Heart valve pathology
- ☐ Enlargement of the heart
- ☐ Any amount of dead cardiac tissue
- ☐ Arrhythmias of the heart
- ☐ Palpitations unrelated to panic attacks

GENERAL MEDICAL

- ☐ Sleep medications take 90-120 minute to take effect instead of 30 minutes
- ☐ Insomnia [If profound fatigue is present, this might not apply]

- ☐ A temperature under 98.3 in a sick person. A temperature under 99.0 if Lyme disease or Babesia is also present
- ☐ An uncomfortable infection in the body with no discernible cause
- ☐ Gastroesophageal reflux disease (GERD)
- ☐ Diarrhea
- ☐ Colitis or an inflammation of the colon
- ☐ Liver enlargement with no clear cause
- ☐ Blood vessel proliferation or increased numbers in any internal organs
- ☐ Lesions or wounds with no clear cause
- ☐ A sore throat with no other clear reason
- ☐ A persistent sore throat in humidity in excess of 45% [low humidity dries out throat tissue]
- ☐ Gingivitis or bleeding during flossing
- ☐ Unusual discomfort on the soles of the feet especially in the morning
- ☐ Puffy tissue on insole or any part of ankles
- ☐ Ankle "edema" or expanded tissue that does not pit when pressed [because it is expanded tissue and not merely fluid]
- ☐ Bone pain
- ☐ Inflammation of the outer bone surface or osteomyelitis
- ☐ Joint pain [this can be also due to Lyme disease and many other medical problems]

- ☐ Muscle pain [this can be also due to Lyme disease and many other medical problems]
- ☐ Medical problems described as "idiopathic" (of unknown or unclear cause)
- ☐ Presence of two tick or flea infections with two positive tick or flea-borne viruses, bacteria or protozoa.

As previously mentioned, Bartonella has more than 30 published species in public genetic databases and has more vectors than possibly any infection in the world. Therefore, the presence of other infections such as tick-borne viruses, bacteria or protozoa, should raise suspicion. Some of these include Babesia, STARI (Masterson's Disease), Neoehrlichia, Anaplasma, Lyme disease, Mycoplasmas, Q Fever, Rocky Mountain spotted fever (Rickettsia), tick-borne relapsing fever, Tularemia (bacteria), Ehrlichia, Protozoa FL1953, and viruses such as CMV, HHV-6, Coxsackie B Types 1, 2, 3, 4, 5, 6, Parvo B-19 or Powassan.

POSSIBLE LABORATORY FINDINGS

- ☐ IL-6 is very low.
- ☐ IL-1B is very low.
- ☐ TNF-alpha is in lower 10% of normal range.
- ☐ VEGF is above the normal range [however, if Babesia is present or being treated the VEGF will fall into normal or abnormal low levels].
- ☐ X-ray of the bone may show areas of bone loss.
- ☐ Biopsies of lymph nodes are negative for Mycoplasma and no clear evidence of other infections or illnesses are found
- ☐ Biopsies of lymph nodes appearing similar to sarcoidosis

☐ Tissue biopsies which are abnormal but with no clear cause of tissue problems

☐ A swab of a fresh scratch or bite skin lesion is positive for Bartonella.

ENVIRONMENT

☐ Exposure to cats and dogs in excess of very incidental rare contact

☐ **Exposure to cats and dogs** that have been strays or go outside [reviews of hundreds of professional journal articles make this a risk in an unknown percentage]

☐ Ticks or fleas are found on any pet you contact

☐ The patient's **mother** is suspected of having Bartonella based on newer direct and **indirect testing.**

☐ A **sibling, father, spouse or child** with any tick or flea-borne infection who shared with the patient a residence or vacation location with proximity to brush

☐ Outdoor exposure to outdoor environments such as brush, wild grasses, wild streams or woods which happened **without** the use of DEET on skin and Permethrin on all clothing (**It only takes one exposure to get a bite**. If you used protection "most of the time," you were still exposed.)

☐ Exposure to lice

☐ Flea bites or flea exposure

☐ Exposure to pets that are exposed to ticks or fleas

☐ A scratch from a cat

☐ A bite from a cat or dog

- ☐ Exposure to biting flies
- ☐ Hunting, living or vacationing near deer or small mammals
- ☐ Clear exposure to any type of tick. [Bartonella is carried by a huge number of carriers, but for now, the percent that carry Bartonella is not known. Further, the capacity to detect all new species in the vectors or in humans infected does not exist or is not routinely available in direct testing of all human infectious Bartonella organisms in both large or specialty labs].
- ☐ Ticks found on your clothing
- ☐ Ticks found on your skin
- ☐ Ticks found in your home or car, vacation spot or recreation area

If one reads the majority of Bartonella journal articles, it seems clear Bartonella harms the body in hundreds of ways. But for our purposes in diagnosis, the above criteria should be enough to prevent a missed diagnosis. More criteria exist. Certainty claims or criticism about Bartonella positions without reading at least of 1,000 articles is confusing. How is this possible with new Bartonella findings and understandings each month? There are also new species whose genetic sequences show their uniqueness almost every month in public databases. In this spirit, this scale is meant merely to increase suspicion of Bartonella, which is a super stealth infection that takes perhaps fifty days to grow out on some bacteria growth plates, and floats in the blood as it lowers fevers. It also clearly suppresses some key immune system fighting chemicals. Cure claims made without the use of **indirect** testing, markedly documented in superior journals, should be examined further to prove effectiveness.

Dr. Schaller is the author of 30 books and 27 top journal articles. His publications address issues in at least twelve fields of medicine. He has the most recent textbook on Bartonella. He has published on Bartonella under the supervision of the former editor of the *Journal of the American Medical Association (JAMA),* and his entries on multiple tick and flea borne infections, including Bartonella [along with Babesia and Lyme disease] were published in a respected infection textbook endorsed by the NIH Director of Infectious Disease. He has seven texts on tick and flea-borne infections based on his markedly unique full-time research and study practice, which is not limited to either finite traditional or integrative progressive medicine. Dr. Schaller has read on these emerging problems for many years.

The Babesia Checklist

Improving Detection of A Common, Emerging Stealth Infection

James L. Schaller, M.D., M.A.R.

Introduction

Below are examples of signs, symptoms and indirect ways to help increase the diagnosis of Babesia. An examination of public genetic databases shows that well over thirty-five species exist, many of which have variants.

Please note that an unknown percentage of people infected with this single celled parasite have no symptoms, at least for many years.

This checklist is not meant to be used as a definitive tool to diagnose Babesia. It is my expert opinion that no definitive 100% or even 98% accurate tool exists.

My goal is merely to decrease illness in those people who are positive but do not show up as positive on a basic direct test (false negative).

Indeed, it is not uncommon for a patient with Babesia to present with a negative test result over ten times, regardless of the laboratory, and then to show up with a positive on DNA testing when exposed to two or three treatments against protozoa for three days, or to have new conversion from negative to positive antibody testing six weeks after a similar provocation trial.

I do not oppose or endorse such approaches, but feel it necessary to mention that the same outcome has occurred with "Malaria-prevention" treatment. Additionally, there have been instances in which the use of herbs, such as artesunate, for cancer prevention, has resulted in an unintended outcome: the conversion of a Babesia antibody titer from negative to positive.

Having authored four books on the topic of Babesia, I have created this scale based on years of full-time reading and a passion to advance detection. This checklist is meant to prevent false negatives: some patients who appear to be negative may not actually be negative. I have done this because my years of full-time reading and research have shown me that missing this parasite for 5, 10, 30 or 50 years is far more dangerous than careful treatment. Treatment side effects are low if the treatment is started at **20% of the suggested dose.**

I would appeal to you that one cannot be considered an expert in treating this potentially fatal infection by merely reading a few articles or guidelines. Nor is expertise acquired by diagnosing and treating the highly obvious, immensely ill, sickest 1% of patients as the "norm" in Babesia diagnosis. Expertise should require ***at least*** a review of 1500 articles over five years. The fact that parasite textbooks usually offer merely 1-2 pages about this infection shows that it is not mastered or understood even by those interested in parasites.

The cure of Babesia does not fit a set formula, but no one should be hopeless about reaching a full recovery. I have currently started a new, research-based, creative thinking textbook on **optimal Babesia treatments** for publication in 2012. It will discuss familiar treatments and offer ideas to maximize these options, but I will also add discussions on newer options for patients and clinicians who are not satisfied with the current options.

In summary, how can any certain medical or scientific Babesia position exist, when new species, sub-species or variants that infect humans are routinely emerging, and for which there is not even a direct test—regardless of sensitivity?

THE BABESIA CHECKLIST

James Schaller, M.D., M.A.R.

(Please Check Any Symptoms That Apply)

PSYCHIATRIC AND NEUROLOGICAL

☐ Family, friends or others report you look tired or foggy

☐ Slowed thinking

☐ Psychiatric label(s) given to a child or relative for all their troubles when clear medical problems exist as shown by abnormal laboratory results (I am not talking about basic organ failure labs, but the use of ***wide testing which includes inflammation and anti-inflammation chemicals, hormones, nutrient levels, and other immune system chemicals***)

☐ Enlarged lymph nodes (but also in Lyme, Bartonella, other infections, high inflammation, tumors and other diseases)

☐ Brain troubles such as trouble keeping up with past routine life demands, lateness due to trouble with motivation and organization, and trouble with concentration [Any of these would be a positive]

☐ Memory troubles [this is not specific to one infection or one disease process. For example, exposure to indoor mold's biological chemicals can decrease memory within an hour depending on the species mix.]

☐ Profound psychiatric illnesses [this is not limited to a single infection.]

HEART & CIRCULATORY SYSTEM

☐ A sudden loss of blood pressure

- ☐ Transfusions using blood that is not your own
- ☐ Anemia even if a non-infectious cause has been proposed
- ☐ Anemia without a clear explanation
- ☐ Severe chest wall pains
- ☐ A "heart attack" before the age of 55 (when you have three risk factors)
- ☐ A "heart attack" or infarct of the heart before the age of 60 years old, with only one risk factor. [Being male is **considered** a risk factor for many. Men **experience** heart damage sooner than women. Other risk factors include tobacco use or exposure, such as second hand smoke at home, diabetes, high blood pressure, high level of sticky cholesterol such as Lipoprotein (a) or high triglyceride levels, family history of heart attacks, limited physical activity, Obesity (might be defined as wearing pants over 39 inches if you are a man and over 34 inches if you a woman or a body fat or body mass index of 30 or higher), excess anger or routine poor handling of stress, and abuse of stimulant drugs such as cocaine or amphetamines. I would add a homocysteine laboratory level over 10, major depression, no vitamin K2 supplementation, a free dihydrotestosterone in the 10th percentile or lower, fragmented or poor sleep [which increases inflammation], a high C4a RIA, a MMPI in excess of 300 and a low VIP blood level.

MAJOR ORGANS

- ☐ A yellow hue on eyes, hands and skin (jaundice) with no other clear cause
- ☐ An enlarged liver (which sits under your right rib cage)

☐ An enlarged spleen (under your left rib cage). **This is falsely believed to be a common human sign; actually it is very rare.**

☐ A ruptured spleen [rare but it gets fast medical attention and therefore is over-represented in medical articles]

☐ Dark urine [this is rarer than some articles intimate]

☐ An inability to urinate

☐ Shortness of breath [no clear asthma, pneumonia, COPD or other common cause]

☐ Pulmonary edema which is a high amount of fluid in the air sacs of the lungs, which leads to shortness of breath

☐ A stroke of any size or in any organ (the word stroke means tissue is unable to get oxygen). The stroke or infarct can be in the brain, retina, kidney, heart and many other tissues.

☐ An MRI, CT or other imaging study that shows dead tissue in any organ with no known cause

GENERAL MEDICAL

☐ Headaches with no clear cause

☐ Headaches which are hard to control and/or severe

☐ Headaches lasting over three years and which increase in pain despite treatments

☐ Weight gain in clear excess of diet and exercise

☐ Weight loss with reasonable eating and average exercise

☐ Excess fat in lower belly area that is in excess of lifestyle and activity

- ☐ Anorexia or a decrease in appetite
- ☐ Any decrease in appetite
- ☐ A poor appetite
- ☐ Fatigue in excess of that experienced by most people in the same age range
- ☐ Fatigue that produces need for sleep in excess of 8 ½ hours daily
- ☐ Fatigue with ongoing insomnia [consider the possibility of both Bartonella and Babesia in this case]
- ☐ Daytime sleep urgency despite nighttime sleep
- ☐ Night sweats
- ☐ Excessive perspiration during normal daily activity
- ☐ Hot flashes in a normal temperature room
- ☐ Intermittent fever
- ☐ Chills
- ☐ Any fever in excess of three days
- ☐ Spike of a fever over 100.5 after a possible tick bite
- ☐ Listlessness
- ☐ Swelling in limbs and other parts of body
- ☐ Waves of generalized itching [this sign of infection and inflammation is not limited just to Babesia.]
- ☐ Lumps or other types of tissue collection with no clear cause [Other tick and flea-borne infections can also cause these growths.]

- ☐ Wasting muscles
- ☐ The general wasting away of body tissue that is visible
- ☐ Profound bone loss in marked excess of that **expected at given age**
- ☐ Excess breast tissue in a man or boy
- ☐ Random stabbing pains
- ☐ Nausea or vomiting
- ☐ Any enhanced sense: sensitivity to light, touch, smells, taste or sound
- ☐ A sense of imbalance
- ☐ One or more medical problems with unclear cause(s), with changing or contradictory diagnoses, or which are eventually called "idiopathic"
- ☐ Two tick or flea infections with two positive tick or flea-borne viruses, bacteria or protozoa. The presence of other infections such as tick-borne viruses or bacteria raises suspicion of a Babesia infection.
- ☐ The presence of one or more mystery illnesses after an evaluation by three quality physicians

LAB RESULTS

- ☐ Eosinophil Cationic Protein (ECP) level is in top 15% of normal. This is altered in perhaps 15-20% of Babesia patients.
- ☐ The ECP level is above normal. (Other things can increase this lab, but it is an error that a Babesia infection is not on these lists).

- ☐ The ECP level increases 30% or more in response to a protozoa killing medication in serial testing. (This test is about 40-60% sensitive and many patients have no change in this lab even with effective treatment).
- ☐ The ECP level is below detectable levels.
- ☐ Absolute Eosinophils in the low or high range [this is not definitive in any manner, but is a useful tool.]
- ☐ A percentage of Eosinophils in low range or high normal range
- ☐ Very high Eosinophils [rare with Babesia, but other findings suggest other possible causes]
- ☐ A normal or low VEGF lab result in the presence of Bartonella
- ☐ A TNF-alpha in excess of 1.0 in the presence of Bartonella
- ☐ A CD57 or CD57/8 level that drops right after the start of a Babesia treatment, or which falls steadily with ongoing Babesia treatment
- ☐ Hemolytic anemia with lab test showing positive blood products in your urine [this is not a routine finding.]
- ☐ Your clinician understands the use of indirect testing and feels your lab pattern is suggestive of the presence of Babesia. This involves more than an ECP spike.
- ☐ Since direct testing for Babesia by any lab misses many human species and is of variable reliability, and the common presence of Bartonella suppresses some antibody tests, a positive or "indeterminate" is likely a positive. Have you had an "indeterminate" or "borderline" Babesia result?
- ☐ Bilirubin abnormality [elevated in perhaps 5 % of patients]

- ☐ Iron abnormalities in excess of normal [high or low levels. The finding of genetic disease that increases iron pathology does not necessarily rule out this finding. The iron pathology can be genetic or acquired illness plus Babesia [See my HES cancer cure paper in Medscape in which the cancer-like eosinophils were primed by Babesia].

- ☐ After Babesia treatment with clear protozoa killing agents used also to kill malaria, IL-6 moves from very low to an increased level.

- ☐ After Babesia treatment with clear protozoa killing agents used also to kill malaria, IL-1B moves from very low to an increased level.

- ☐ Babesia creates and provokes changes in the human body chemistry. Tests are being designed to identify chemicals only made by Babesia. A sample is Babesia microti secreted antigen 1 (BmSA1).

- ☐ Any positive Epstein-Barr virus over the normal low level. You may have an infection, infections, or inflammation. It is not merely found in Babesia. [This is not a routine cause of fatigue].

- ☐ Autoimmunity testing is positive. This is a stronger positive if there are two autoimmune results. For example, a patient has a positive ANA and has antibodies against their thyroid system.

- ☐ Positive lab or skin testing placing patient's food sensitivity in top 5% of population

- ☐ Elevated monocytes

- ☐ Elevated neutrophils with no clear infection source

- ☐ Elevated C-reactive protein

- ☐ Elevated D-dimer
- ☐ An abnormally high ALT which is a liver enzyme increased by liver trauma, toxins or infections such as Babesia [a rare finding].
- ☐ Lymphocytopenia—low lymphocytes which are a type of infection-fighting white blood cell
- ☐ Thrombocytopenia—platelet number under 50,000
- ☐ A high lactate dehydrogenase or LDH. This enzyme measures tissue damage particularly found in the heart, liver, kidney, skeletal muscle, brain, blood cells and lungs.

REACTION OR CHANGES IN BODY

- ☐ React to any derivative of Artemisia (Sweet Wormwood). *Note: the reaction does not need to last more than a day and any immediate stomachaches or loose stools do not apply.
- ☐ React to a malaria drug. For example, ativoquone (Mepron), proguanil alone or with ativoquone (Malarone), artesunate, day 1-3 of artemesinin, a new high dose of artemesinin Day 1-2, artemeter, Alinia, clindamycin, quinine or azithromycin at 2,000 mg/day orally or at any dose IV for five straight days. (It requires profound wisdom for a clinician to distinguish between a side effect and a reaction caused by an effective Babesia treatment. For example, insomnia caused by the synthetic drug Larium is meaningless, since Larium has this as a side effect in uninfected patients. But fatigue, insomnia or severe headache resulting from a teaspoon of ativoquone (Mepron) on day one are very suspicious symptoms for a known protozoan like Babesia or Malaria or other similar infections that are newly identified genetically).
- ☐ Mood changes with any herb or drug that kills protozoa like Babesia, with the exception of Larium

☐ Muscle aches or joint aches/pain, especially worse after use of a protozoa killing medicine such as proquanil, Alinia, ativoquone, clindamycin, or one of many new emerging progressive natural medicine or synthetic malaria drug treatments

☐ Insomnia after taking a malaria killing herb or drug

☐ Anxiety and/or depression after taking a malaria killing herb or drug

☐ Rage or temporary personality regression right after use of a malaria killing herb or medication, e.g., ativoquone, Malarone, proguanil, artesunate, day 1-3 of artemesinin, artemeter, Alinia, clindamycin or azithromycin at 2,000 mg/day orally or at any dose IV for five straight days.

ENVIRONMENT

☐ Pets, farm animals or local relatives with ANY **clinical symptoms** of a tick-borne virus, bacteria or protozoa infection without a clear diagnosis

☐ The patient's **mother** is suspected of having or has been diagnosed with Babesia, STARI (Masterson's Disease), Neoehrlichia, Anaplasma, Lyme disease, Mycoplasmas, Q Fever, Rocky Mountain spotted fever (Rickettsia), tick-borne relapsing fever, Tularemia (bacteria), Ehrlichia, Protozoa FL1953, or viruses such as CMV, HHV-6, Coxsackie B Types 1, 2, 3, 4, 5, 6, Parvo B-19 or Powassan.

☐ **A sibling, father, spouse or child** with any tick borne infection who shared a residence or vacation with proximity to brush (wooded area)

☐ Exposure to outdoor environments with brush, wild grasses, wild streams, golf courses or woods ***in excess of ten minutes in any location lived in or visited***

- ☐ **Pet(s) or family animals** of any type, e.g., horses, have had outdoor exposures to areas with brush, wild grasses, wild streams or woods. If the pets were animals such as dogs, which can be given anti-tick and flea treatments, were these animals always ***on schedule*** with these treatments?

- ☐ Clear exposure to ticks in your current or past homes

- ☐ Clear exposure to ticks during vacations or other travels

- ☐ Have you ever had any type of tick bite?

- ☐ Have you ever found a tick on your clothing?

- ☐ Have you ever found a tick on your body?

- ☐ Have you been with others at a location in which they had ticks on their clothing or skin?

- ☐ Sexual contact is a debated form of communication of some tick and flea borne infections. I have no position. Isolation in a body fluid does not mean that is a route to spread the infection. If you and your healer feel this is a possible route of infection, has the patient had intimate contact with the sharing of body fluids with an infected person?

- ☐ You live in a state that has reports of any tick-borne infection in over 40 people. [Currently, this would usually be Lyme disease only].

- ☐ You live next to a state that has reports of any tick-borne infection in over 60 people. [Currently, this would usually be Lyme disease only].

- ☐ Many small mammals live near your home, exercise location, vacation locations or work.

A WORD ON MANUAL BLOOD EXAMINATIONS

No blood smear will be positive for Babesia unless you have a profound number of infected red blood cells. This is very rare. Therefore, **no blood smear should be considered negative unless it has been examined for at least thirty minutes.** While a 2-3 minute exam of large white blood cells may be fully sufficient to identify cancers and other diseases, a search for over eighty Babesia red blood cell presentations under 1000x, as found in my book, *Hematology Forms of Babesia,* requires at least thirty minutes. Unfortunately, in patients positive for Babesia, routine manual red blood smear exams with a clear request to look for Babesia under a microscope at 1,000x magnification have missed the Babesia at least 98% of the time. In papers reporting clearly visualized Babesia in blood smears the patients tend to have immense infection, i.e., over 3% of red blood cells are infected.

However, if one privately contracts with a microbiologist, pathologist or can get a lab director to allow their staff to spend the extra time, the positive results on the blood smear increase with clearly positively infected patients. I know most laboratories are very overworked, but the notion that a blood slide is going to show an obvious tetrad or a classic X pattern is an error. Using slides from respected national or state sources, I found only by very careful exam, over fifty presentations of Babesia that are usually missed. Indeed, in my textbook on Babesia images most of the shapes had never been published. No one in history had ever taken the time to look carefully at 200 slides and record each unique shape. It is fairly stunning to write this and confirms that many tick and flea infections are clearly emerging and not yet mastered.

Please appreciate that stains help define whether a substance is what it appears to be. For example, some in the alternative medicine school feel that Candida is a bad presence in the intestines and feel it often gets into the blood through defects in the intestinal wall. While Candida is not a good presence for the intestine, I have found that some blood samples with items that look significantly like parts of Candida do not stain for cellulose and other components of yeasts. My point is that in the last ten years, in discussions or study, excellent pathologists and microbiologists have shown me the clear reason humanity has developed highly sophisticated staining techniques—they can be diagnostic and very cost effective. And some medical scientists are adding new technology to Babesia identification (discussed in my *Babesia 2009 Update* and my *Hematology of Babesia* text).

Babesia is an emerging infection. Any certainty claims or criticism about Babesia positions without extensive research and over 200 hours of reading is premature. Again, new Babesia species are emerging every one to four months. Indeed, even a new protozoan has been found that looks like Babesia under a high powered microscope, but when it is genetically sequenced it is not Babesia or immature malaria, which can look similar. It is a new infection and is presently called FL1953 and was genetically sequenced by Dr. Ellis and Dr. Fry. It looks like Babesia, but is not Babesia genetically.

Therefore, since human Babesia is a new emerging illness, this scale is meant merely to increase awareness of Babesia, an infection that can kill patients of any age. Writings in the past fifteen years have either seen Babesia as a mere "co-infection" or a footnote of a spirochete infection [i.e., Lyme]. Anything that can hide for a couple of decades, and then possibly kill you with a clot in your heart, brain or lungs or by other means, is not a casual infection.

Babesia cure claims should be made with the use of indirect testing birthed from extracts of superior journals read a minimum of five years. Currently, these many well-established indirect lab test patterns are not used or understood by immensely busy and smart clinicians working full-time. While this is fully understandable, I hope it may change in the coming decade.

Dr. Schaller is the author of 30 books and 27 top journal articles. His publications address issues in at least twelve fields of medicine.

He has published the most recent four textbooks on Babesia.

He has published on Babesia as a cancer primer under the supervision of the former editor of the *Journal of the American Medical Association (JAMA),* and his entries on multiple tick and flea-borne infections, including Babesia [along with Bartonella and Lyme disease], were published in a respected infection textbook endorsed by the NIH Director of Infectious Disease.

Dr. Schaller has produced seven texts on tick and flea-borne infections based on his markedly unique full-time reading and study practice, which is not limited to either finite traditional or integrative progressive medicine. With a physician's medical license, he has been able to sort through many truth claims by ordering lab testing. He does not casually follow the dozens of yearly truth claims, without indirect testing laboratory proof. He has read full-time on these emerging problems for many years. He is rated a TOP and BEST physician (in the top 5 percent of doctors) by both physician peers and patients.

LYME DISEASE SYMPTOM CHECKLIST

James Schaller, M.D., M.A.R.

INTRODUCTION

The following checklist is not meant to be complete or authoritative. Information about Lyme disease is constantly emerging and changing. Therefore any checklist is intended for use as a starting point. In traditional medicine, a physician performs a complete history and physical. Labs and studies **assist** in clarifying the differential diagnosis. In Lyme disease, much debate exists about laboratory kits, the alteration of kits to have fewer possible bands, and which labs are optimally sensitive and specific. This checklist is not intended to address that issue or treatment.

Over 200 animals carry the Ixodes tick, which is the most commonly known insect spreading Lyme disease. With so many vectors, the underlying assumption behind this checklist is that Lyme is not rare in North America, Europe, South America, Russia, Africa or Asia.

We know Lyme disease is highly under-reported. One study showed only 1 in 40 family doctors reported it.

Immediately upon biting, the tick transmits a pain killer, antihistamine and an anti-coagulant. Based on animal studies, it is also possible the bulls-eye rash is less common than assumed, in part because injections of spirochete related material in laboratory animals only show a rash with the **second** injection. With this background, I would appeal, that if a young or middle aged adult experiences a bite, and has profound symptoms, is it possible this was a small number of infectious particles igniting a larger number from 2, 5 or 20 years earlier? I am not asking for an answer, just for the possibility to be considered.

This checklist is offered with the sincere wish that others will improve on it. It is this author's personal belief that tick and flea-borne infection medicine is as specialized as HIV and Hepatitis medical science and treatment.

Some of the checklist materials might be new to you, which underscores the need for another scale to add to the ones currently in existence. This list is based on a massive review of thousands of papers over a decade of full-time reading, 2012 science revelations, and/or massive chart reviews. Since modern Lyme disease seems to focus on tick-borne disease and other laboratory testing, we will start with lab testing considerations. If a lab test has a value or a percentage, the numbers chosen are intended to avoid missing those positive patients who otherwise would be overlooked. The concern is about physicians and other health care workers not treating an infected patient, who over time can experience disability or even death at a frequency that is impossible to determine.

THE LYME DISEASE CHECKLIST

James Schaller, M.D., M.A.R.

(Please Check Any Symptoms That Apply)

LABORATORY TESTING — INDIRECT AND DIRECT

- ☐ Vitamin D level is in the lowest 20%. If you supplement, it should be in top 50%.
- ☐ CD57 or CD58 is in the lowest 20th percentile.
- ☐ Free testosterone is in 10th percentile or below.
- ☐ In 5% of patients the testosterone or free testosterone is over the normal range.
- ☐ DHEA is in lower 20%. Or rarely is it fully over the top level.
- ☐ Free dihydrotestosterone is in the lowest 20th percentile or well over the normal range.
- ☐ Epstein Barr Virus is abnormal in any measure. [This virus is believed to be positive over normal positive levels in the presence of infections or high inflammation.]
- ☐ On the Western Blot, IgG or IgM any ***species specific*** band at any blood level, e.g., 18, 21, 23, 30, 31, 34, 37, 39, 83, 93.
- ☐ A free T3 level under 2.8 [the normal bottom range in 1990 was 2.6; the influx of large numbers of elderly patients reset the healthy "normal" range].
- ☐ Positive for viruses such as CMV, HHV-6, Coxsackie B Types 1, 2, 3, 4, 5, 6, Parvo B-19 or Powassan virus
- ☐ Positive for Mycoplasma, e.g. mycoplasma pneumonia

- ☐ The patient is positive for infections other than **routine** Lyme, [that is **Borrelia burgdorferi sensu stricto,** Borrelia **afzelii** and Borrelia **garinii**]. Some of the other infections also carried by infectious ticks, fleas or other vectors include Babesia (duncani, microti or other), Anaplasma (HGA), Ehrlichia (various species/strains), Neoehrlichia, Rocky Mountain or other Spotted Fevers, Brucellosis, Q-fever, STARI (Master's Disease), Malaria, and Bartonella [e.g., B. henselae, B. quintana, B. elizabethae and B. melophagi]. Once tests are commercially available for testing all forms of protozoa affecting humans, including FL1953, all Bartonella species, and Borrelia miyamotoi and other Lyme species, reporting should increase.

- ☐ IL-B is in lowest 10th percentile.

- ☐ IL-6 is in lowest 10th percentile.

- ☐ TNF-alpha is under 2, or in lowest 20th percentile.

- ☐ A WBC count was, or is, under 4.5.

- ☐ Eosinophil level in the CBC manual exam is either at 0-1 or 6-7.

- ☐ Total manual Eosinophil level is 140 or less.

- ☐ X-ray or other study shows cartilage defects in excess of injury or age median.

- ☐ If a full auto-immunity panel is run with at least eight different tests, two are positive; for example, you have a positive anti-gliadin and a positive thyroid peroxidase.

- ☐ Positive or near positive (borderline) ELISA, PCR, or a positive tissue biopsy; or a tick from your body is positive for Lyme or other tick infection

- ☐ Lab tests show high inflammation, e.g., a high C4a, elevated cholesterol and C-peptide. These are never specific just for Lyme.
- ☐ Lab tests show a MSH level under 30 [the reference range of 0-40 is due to the increase of very sick patients tested, and 40-85 is a better reference range which was used before the flood of the sick reset the range of normal]. MSH is an anti-inflammatory hormone.
- ☐ VIP is under 20. This is an anti-inflammation chemical.

BODY EXAMINATION RESULTS

- ☐ Weight loss or gain in excess of 20 pounds in 12 weeks
- ☐ A round or oval rash with a dark center was or is present in a loose "bulls-eye pattern" or other size and shape rashes that have no other cause after exposure to ticks and vectors
- ☐ Healing is slow after scratches or surgery. For example, after a cat scratch, flea bite or tick bite the mark is still visible later.
- ☐ Skin on arms, hands or feet has a texture like rice paper.
- ☐ Clear reaction and effect is seen with antibiotic treatment. Specifically, a marked improvement or worsening of a serious medical problem or function is observed with a spirochete killing treatment, e.g., doxycycline, tetracycline, minocycline, any penicillin such as amoxicillin, azithromycin, clarithromycin or cefuroxime.
- ☐ Presence of skin tags, red papules of any size, excess blood vessels compared to peers, and stretch marks with color or in significant excess of peers.
- ☐ Moles and raised or hard plaques in excess of the few on normal skin

- ☐ Areas of skin with ulcerations such as those seen in syphilis, but at any location on the body
- ☐ Areas of clear hypo-pigmentation and hyper-pigmentation
- ☐ Positive ACA (Acrodermatitis chronica atrophicans) which is a sign of long term untreated Lyme disease. Some report ACA begins as a reddish-blue patch of discolored skin, often of the hands or feet. It may include the back in some patients. The lesion slowly atrophies over months to years, with many developing skin that is thin, dry, hairless, wrinkled and abnormally colored. The color of the extremities such as hands and feet can be red, dark red, brown, dark blue or purple.

Sample Neurological Exam

- ☐ Patient's short-term memory is poor. For example, if asked to recall these numbers—23, 5, 76, 43 and 68—the patient cannot recall them.
- ☐ Patient cannot reverse four numbers, so if given—18, 96, 23 and 79—the patient cannot do it.
- ☐ If asked to subtract 17 from 120, (college graduate), it cannot be done in a timely manner. If a high school graduate, subtract 7 from 100 and continue to subtract by 7 four times in 20 seconds.
- ☐ Light headedness upon standing quickly in excess of peers, and with no clear cause
- ☐ Dizziness unrelated to position
- ☐ Dizziness made worse by Lyme killing antibiotics

- ☐ Trouble doing a nine step **heel to toe straight line walk test** with fingers slightly in pockets [The patient should not sway or need their hands pulled out to prevent a fall]. In patients with past experience in skating, skiing, dance or ballet this should be ***very easy*** and is rarely a challenge to such people. If it is not easy, it is suspicious medically, but not only for Lyme disease.

- ☐ Trouble performing a one leg lift, in which one leg is lifted 15 inches off the ground in front of you, as you count, e.g., "one Mississippi, two Mississippi, etc."

- ☐ Positive nystagmus [your eye jerks when you look right or left]

PATIENT'S REPORTED PHYSICAL HISTORY

Psychiatric & Neurological

- ☐ Mild to severe neurological disorders or psychiatric disorders

- ☐ A very profound neurological disease which does not clearly fit the labs, studies and course of the illness

- ☐ A moderate or severe medical, psychiatric or neurological illness. [Many severe disorders can be associated with spirochetes such as those causing syphilis, and some propose that Lyme is also related to a well-known serious brain disease.]

- ☐ Severe medical, psychiatric or neurology illness with uncommon features, such as Parkinson's disease, appearing at a young age

- ☐ Facial paralysis (Bell's palsy)

- ☐ Personality has changed negatively and significantly for no clear reason.

- ☐ Psychosis at any age, but especially after 40 years of age when ***usually*** it would have already manifested itself
- ☐ Severe anxiety
- ☐ Mania or profound rage
- ☐ Depression with minimal genetic risk
- ☐ Depression or anxiety that did not exist when you were less than 25 years of age
- ☐ Irritability
- ☐ Any one of the following: paranoia, dementia, schizophrenia, bipolar disorder, panic attacks, major depression, anorexia nervosa or obsessive-compulsive disorder
- ☐ Adult onset ADHD/ADD [Primary psychiatric biological ADD or ADHD is present at 7 years of age. Adult onset may be a sign of a medical condition.]
- ☐ Increased verbal or physical fighting with others
- ☐ Functioning at work or in parenting is at least 20% reduced
- ☐ Patience and relational skills are decreased by 20% or more
- ☐ A mild to profound decrease of insight, i.e., an infected patient does not see their decreased function, failed treatment or personality change
- ☐ A new eccentric rigidity to hearing new medical or other important information
- ☐ Difficulty thinking or concentrating
- ☐ Poor memory and reduced ability to concentrate
- ☐ Increasingly difficult to recall names of people or things

- ☐ Difficulty speaking or reading
- ☐ Difficulty finding the words to express what you want to say
- ☐ Inability to learn new information as well as in the past [receptive learning]
- ☐ Repeating stories or forgetting information told to close relations, such as a spouse, roommate, sibling, best friend or parent
- ☐ Confusion without a clear reason
- ☐ An addiction that results in relapse in spite of sincere, reasonable and serious efforts to stop
- ☐ Fatigue in excess of normal, or fatigue that is getting worse
- ☐ Trouble sleeping including mild to severe insomnia and disrupted sleep
- ☐ Sleep in excess of 9 hours a day or night, or sleeping in excess of 9 hours every day if allowed
- ☐ Trouble falling asleep
- ☐ Trouble staying asleep [Taking a 5 minute bathroom break does not count]

Major Organs

- ☐ Gastritis or stomach sensitivity not caused by H. Pylori
- ☐ Intestinal troubles that are unable to be fully managed and/or which have no clear diagnosis
- ☐ Nausea without a clear reason
- ☐ Ear problems such as pain or increased ear "pressure"

☐ ***Any trouble*** with the senses (vision, sound, touch, taste or smell). The use of corrective lenses or contacts does not count, unless the prescription is changed more than expected.

☐ Buzzing or ringing in ears

☐ Double vision, floaters, dry eyes, or other vision trouble

☐ Conjunctivitis (pinkeye) or occasional damage to deep tissue in the eyes

☐ Bladder dysfunction of any kind

☐ Treatment resistant interstitial cystitis

☐ Blood clots fast when you get a cut, or you have a diagnosed problem with clotting. This may also be seen in blood draws where blood draw needle clots when blood is being removed. If on a blood thinner, blood thinness level goes up and down too much.

☐ Cardiac impairment

☐ Chest pain with all labs and studies in normal range

☐ Occasional rapid heartbeats (palpitations)

☐ Heart block/heart murmur

☐ Heart valve prolapse

☐ Shortness of breath with no clear cause on pulmonary function tests, examination, lab testing, X-rays, MRI's, etc.

☐ Air hunger or feelings of shortness of breath

Skin

☐ Numbness, tingling, burning, or shock sensations in an area of skin

- ☐ One or more troublesome skin sensations that move over months or years and do not always stay in one location
- ☐ Rash or rashes without a simple and obvious cause
- ☐ Rashes that persist despite treatment
- ☐ Eccentric itching with no clear cause
- ☐ Hair loss with no clear cause

Musculoskeletal

- ☐ Muscle pain or cramps
- ☐ Muscle spasms
- ☐ Muscle wasting without a clear cause
- ☐ Trouble with your jaw muscle(s) or joint insomnia (TMJ)
- ☐ Joint defects in one joint with no clear cause if 20 or younger
- ☐ Joint defects in two joints or more if 35 or younger
- ☐ Joint defects in three or more locations if younger than 55 with no clear trauma
- ☐ Swelling or pain (inflammation) in the joints [Most patients ***never*** have joint disease.]
- ☐ Joint pain that shifts location
- ☐ Neck stiffness
- ☐ Chronic arthritis with or without episodes of swelling, redness, and fluid buildup

General Medical

- ☐ Gaining or losing weight in a manner clearly inconsistent with diet and exercise
- ☐ New or more food allergies than ten years ago
- ☐ Feel worse after eating breads, pasta or sweets
- ☐ No longer tolerate or enjoy alcohol
- ☐ Anti-histamines are bothersome, more so than in the past.
- ☐ Reaction to medications is excessive (you are very "sensitive" to medications)
- ☐ Your response to antibiotics is significantly positive and you feel more functional, ***or you have the opposite reaction*** and feel worse, feeling ill, fatigued or agitated.
- ☐ Chronic pain in excess of what seems reasonable
- ☐ Nerve pain without a clear cause
- ☐ Sensitivity to lights, sounds, touch, smell or unusual tastes
- ☐ Sensitivity to cleaning chemicals, fragrances and perfumes
- ☐ Headaches that do not respond fully to treatment, or which are getting worse
- ☐ New allergies or increased allergies over those of your peers
- ☐ Any autoimmunity--Lyme and other tick infections, over many years, increase inflammation and decrease anti-inflammation chemicals. We believe this leads to increased food sensitivities, increased autoimmunity and a heightened sensitivity to various chemicals and medications.
- ☐ Day time sweats

- ☐ Night time sweats
- ☐ Chills
- ☐ Flu-like symptoms
- ☐ Abnormal menstrual cycle
- ☐ Decreased or increased libido
- ☐ Increased motion sickness
- ☐ Fainting
- ☐ A spinning sensation or vertigo
- ☐ Illnesses that come and go and decrease functioning with no certain cause
- ☐ Serious illnesses that undermine function with no clear cause, and which affect more than one body organ
- ☐ An abnormal lab result, physical exam finding or illness that is given many diagnoses or has no clear cause

ENVIRONMENT

- ☐ Someone in your neighborhood within 400 yards in any direction of your dwelling has been diagnosed with a tick borne infection [This includes vacation locations].
- ☐ You have someone living with you with any type of tick-borne infection—this assumes they were not merely tested for one infection. [It is not proven that the small Lyme-carrying ticks only carry Lyme, and it is possible some carry other infections without carrying Lyme at all.
- ☐ You have removed any ticks ***from your body*** in your lifetime at any location.

- ☐ You have removed ticks ***from your clothing*** in your lifetime at any location.
- ☐ After a tick or bug bite, you had a fever for at least 48 hours.
- ☐ After a tick or bug bite, you were ill.
- ☐ Grew up or played in areas with many small wild mammals
- ☐ When you are in a room that has visible mold or smells like mold and you start to feel ill, you do not return to your baseline health in 24 hours.
- ☐ Any discomfort ***within two minutes*** of being in a musty or moldy location. This may be a sign of chronic untreated infection, because a mere 30 inhalations of mold debris causes systemic effects in your body
- ☐ ***Pets or farm animals*** positive with ANY tick borne virus, bacteria or protozoa, or clinical symptoms without a clear diagnosis or cause
- ☐ The patient's **mother** is suspected of having or has been diagnosed with Babesia, Ehrlichia, Rocky Mountain Spotted Fever, Anaplasma, Lyme, Bartonella or other tick borne disease based on newer direct and indirect testing, or clinical signs and symptoms.
- ☐ **A sibling, father, spouse or child** with any tick-borne infection
- ☐ **Casual or work-related exposure to outdoor environments** with brush, wild grasses, wild streams or woods (Examples- golf courses, parks, gardens, river banks, swamps, etc.)
- ☐ Pets, e.g., horses, dogs or cats, have had **outdoor exposures** to areas such as brush, wild grasses, wild streams or woods.
- ☐ You played in grass in the past.

- ☐ You have been bitten by fleas.
- ☐ You have been scratched by a cat or dog.

FINAL WORDS

Some of the above listed signs and symptoms fit other infections that may be more common than Lyme disease. Unfortunately, the research and experience indicating diverse infections carried by the Ixodes and other ticks is ignored so a small number of symptoms and signs were added to this checklist. Further, "testing" usually involves one test for a mono-infection—Borrelia or Lyme. Ticks and other vectors should never be assumed to carry only Lyme disease.

Please note that when we are talking about the Ixodes tick we are ***not*** referring to this as a "deer tick" since it has over 200 vectors (Ostfeld). **Many of the tick reduction options presently suggested are not successful in accomplishing their goals.** Reducing deer populations, once thought to reduce tick populations and incidence of Lyme disease, may simply increase tick numbers in mammals and other carriers that live closer to humans.

All healers have their familiar way of thinking, testing and treating. Kuhn has shown we are all biased and struggle to be objective…and fail. Certainty is simply impossible in medical science. Further, tick and flea infections have almost infinite pathological effects because the human body and these clusters of infections are so complex. I have not suggested a grid or a set number of symptoms, because one would not fit this list. Simply, the goal of this checklist is to have you think broadly.

You cannot use this checklist to diagnose Lyme disease or to rule it out.

A Lyme checklist is very medically important, since it is still an emerging illness and can sometimes disable or increase mortality risk in patients of any age if not diagnosed and treated early in the infection.

Writings in the past fifteen years have either viewed Babesia and Bartonella as mere "co-infections," or a footnote of a spirochete infection [i.e., Lyme]. Either infection can hide for decades, and then possibly disable or kill a person by causing a clot, heart arrhythmia or by other means.

The detection of Lyme from stained tissue samples or blood is very difficult. Currently, the well-established indirect lab test patterns presented are not used or understood by all health care professionals. While this is fully understandable, I hope it may change in the coming decade. Tick infections have ***systemic impacts*** on the body, and are not limited to effects reported in journal articles, a few books or any national or international guidelines.

Dr. Schaller has published the four most recent textbooks on Babesia and the only recent textbook in any language on Bartonella. His most recent book on Lyme, Babesia and Bartonella includes a "researchers only" list of over 2,600 references considered to be **a start** for basic education in tick infection medicine.

He published articles on both Babesia as a cancer primer and Bartonella as a profound psychiatric disease under the supervision of the former editor of the *Journal of the American Medical Association (JAMA)*. He also published entries on multiple tick and flea-borne infections, including Babesia, Bartonella and Lyme disease, in a respected infection textbook endorsed by the NIH Director of Infectious Disease.

Dr. Schaller is the author of seven texts on tick and flea-borne infections. He is rated a BEST physician, an honor that is awarded to only 1 in 20 physicians by physician peers. He is also rated a TOP physician by patients, again ranking in the top 5 percent of physicians.

This form may not be altered if it is printed or posted, in any manner, without written permission. It can be printed for free to assist in diagnostic reflections, as long as no line is redacted or altered, including the introduction or final paragraphs. Dr. Schaller does not claim that this is a flawless or final form, and defers all diagnostic decisions to your licensed health professional.

Dr. Schaller has been published in:

Journal of the American Medical Association

Journal of Clinical Neuroscience

Medscape (Academic Journal of WebMD)

Journal of the American Society of Child and Adolescent Psychiatry

American Journal of Psychiatry

European Journal of Child and Adolescent Psychiatry

Compounding Pharmaceuticals: Triad

Fleming Revell Press (Four Languages)

Internal Medicine News

Family Practice News

Spire Mass Market Books

Internet Journal of Family Medicine

Greenwood Press

Child and Adolescent Psychiatry Drug Alerts

Hope Academic Press

Clinical Psychiatry News

Psychiatric Drug Alerts

Townsend Journal

OB/GYN News

AMA News

Currents

A Sample of Other Books by Dr. Schaller

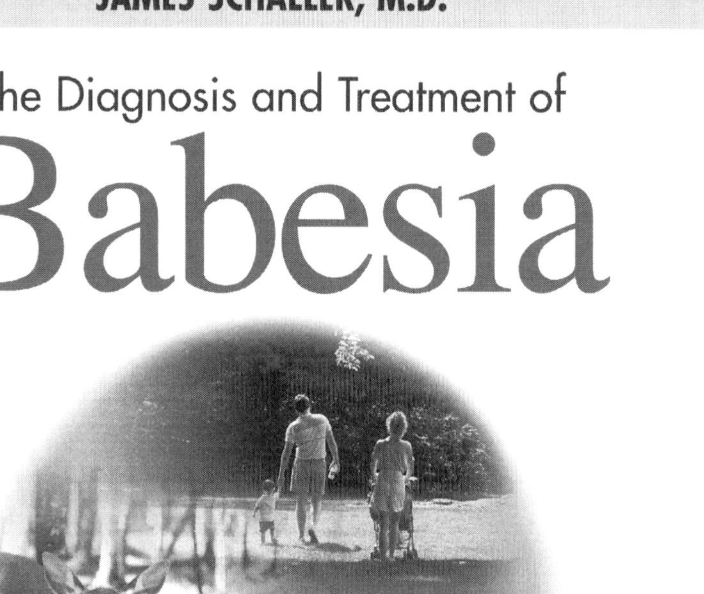

This large textbook is clear and easy to read. It is really three books. While some points are partially outdated since 2006, much would be considered new to most readers.

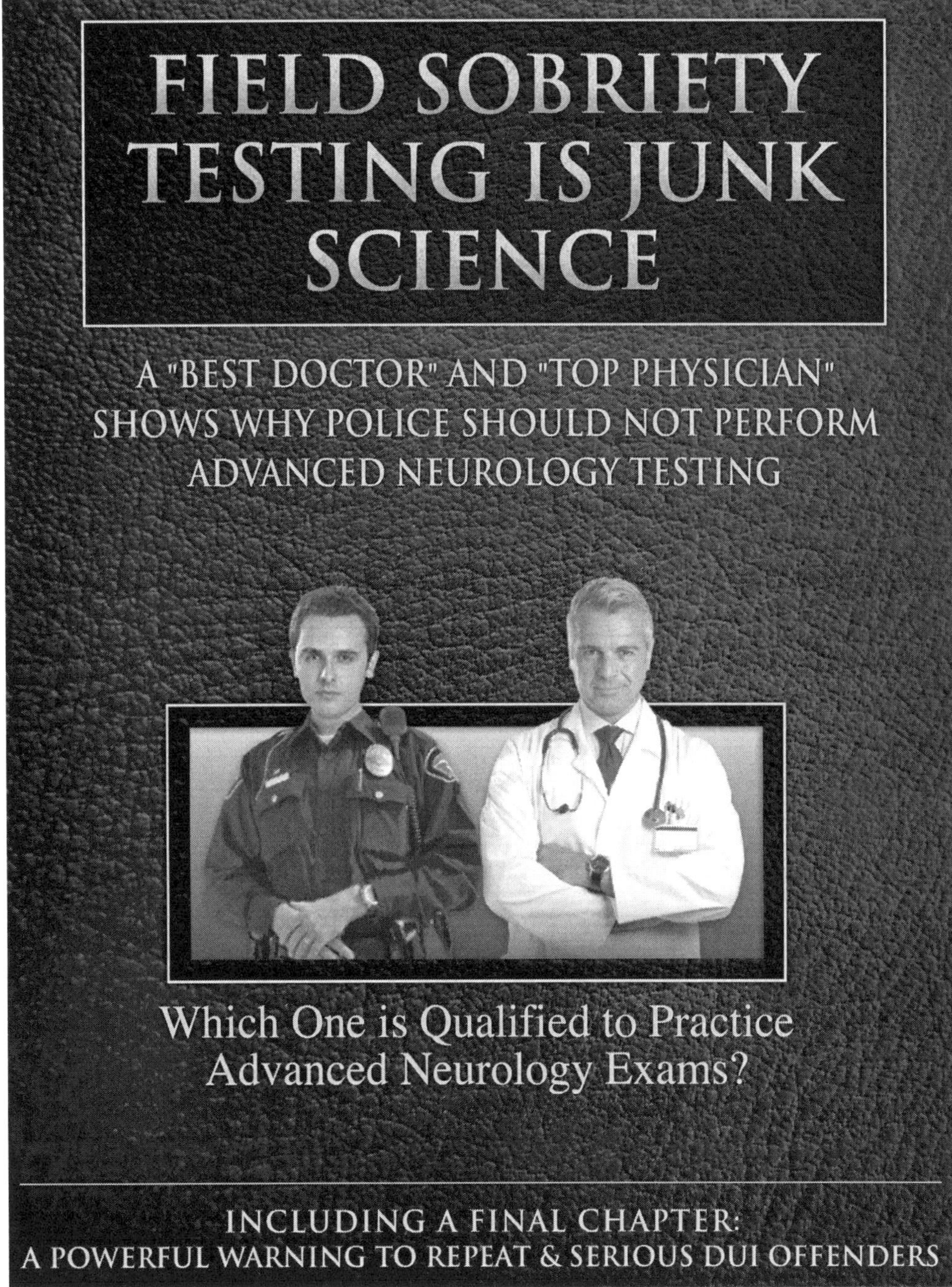

It appeals to all peace officers, legislatures, and concerned citizens to rethink the science of these super medical examinations which help save lives, **but also often allow for many to be placed under arrest for over 500 medical problems.**

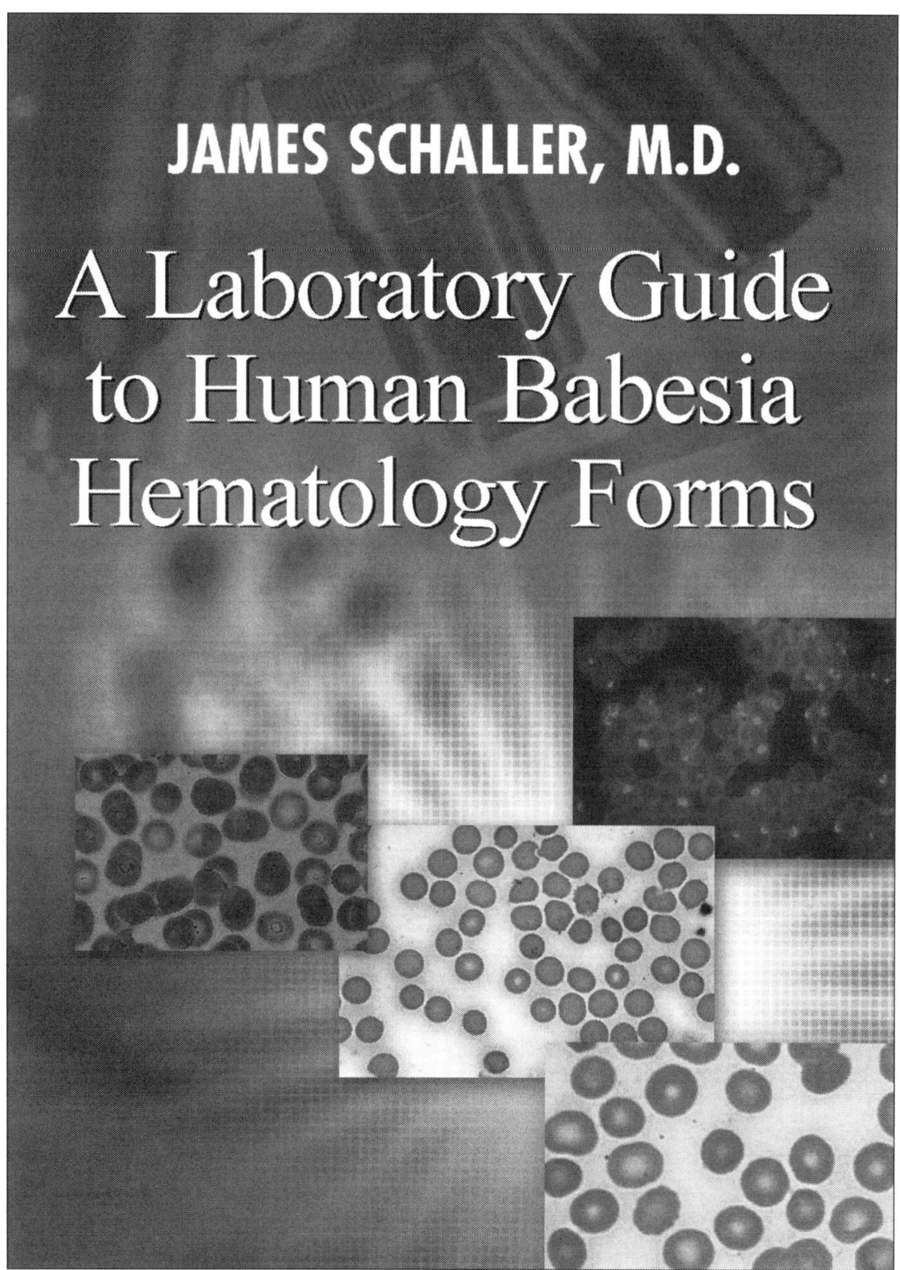

The only hematology book exclusively dedicated to Babesia.

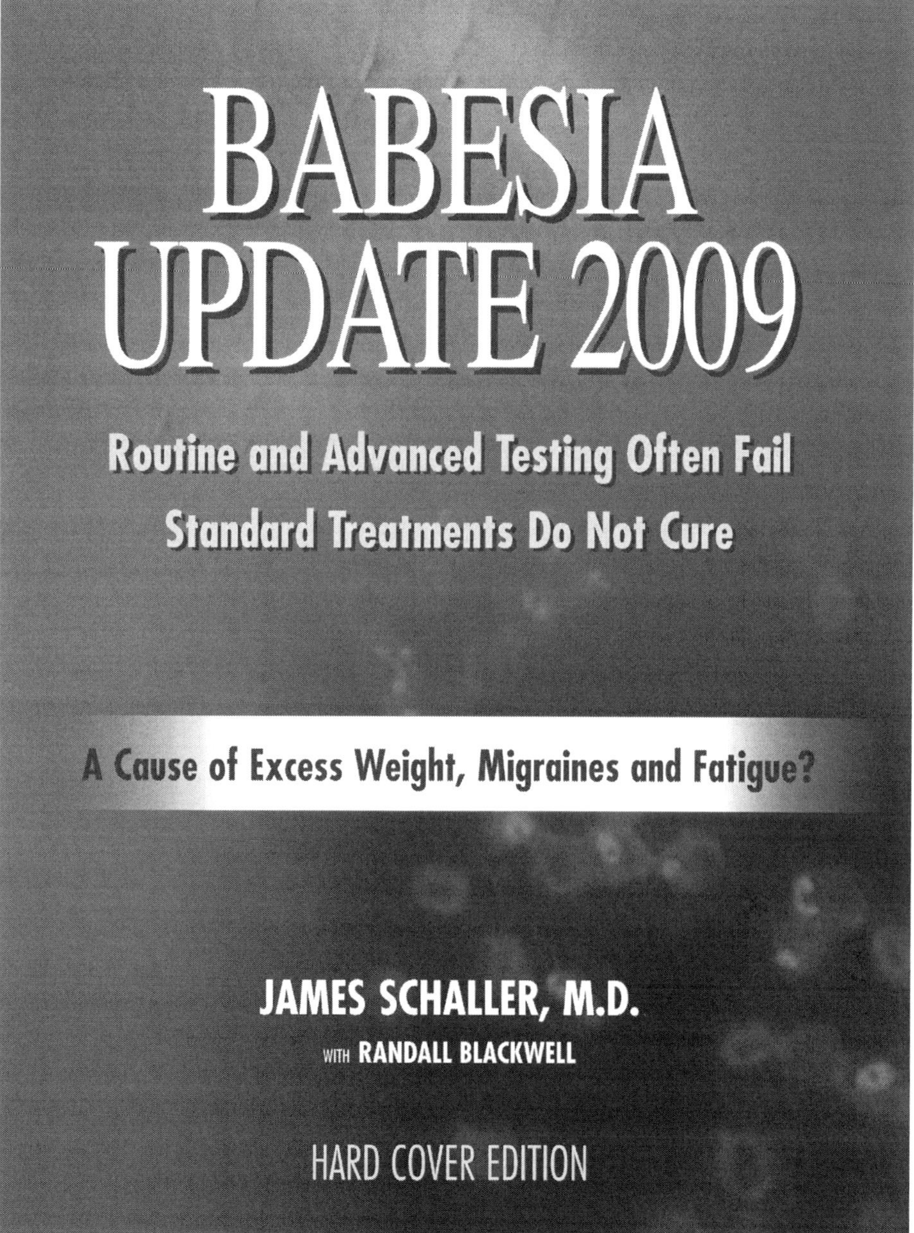

A book with advanced research based information, that moves Babesia medicine into a new decade. It presents highly practical information on ways to detect Babesia that are not mere IgM/G titer tests. Learn how to detect new species being discovered routinely and which seriously undermine function. This text also discusses why some individuals do not experience the easy and fast cure promised in other writings.

JAMES SCHALLER, M.D.

The Diagnosis, Treatment and Prevention of

Bartonella

Atypical Bartonella Treatment Failures and 40 Hypothetical Physical Exam Findings

Bartonella diagnosis is very complex. This current text creatively uses a new set of tools to assist in diagnosis based on solid research of blood vessel and skin augmentation chemicals created by Bartonella. It literally creates a new Bartonella physical exam. This book helps with limited basic lab testing, and **prevents the use of routinely relapsing or poor treatments promoted in both traditional and integrative medicine.** No other book on this topic is based on over a thousand top research articles, and no one has published anything remotely close to replacing this work in over five years.

When Traditional Medicine Fails...

YOUR GUIDE TO MOLD TOXINS

Gary Rosen, Ph.D. & James Schaller, M.D.

- WHAT THEY ARE
- WHO THEY HURT
- AND WHAT YOU CAN DO TO RECLAIM YOUR CHILD'S HEALTH, LEARNING AND BEHAVIOR

Includes Home Detox Program

Dr. Schaller is a Certified Mold Investigator and a Certified Mold Remediator. Here is a practical and readable mold mycotoxin book.

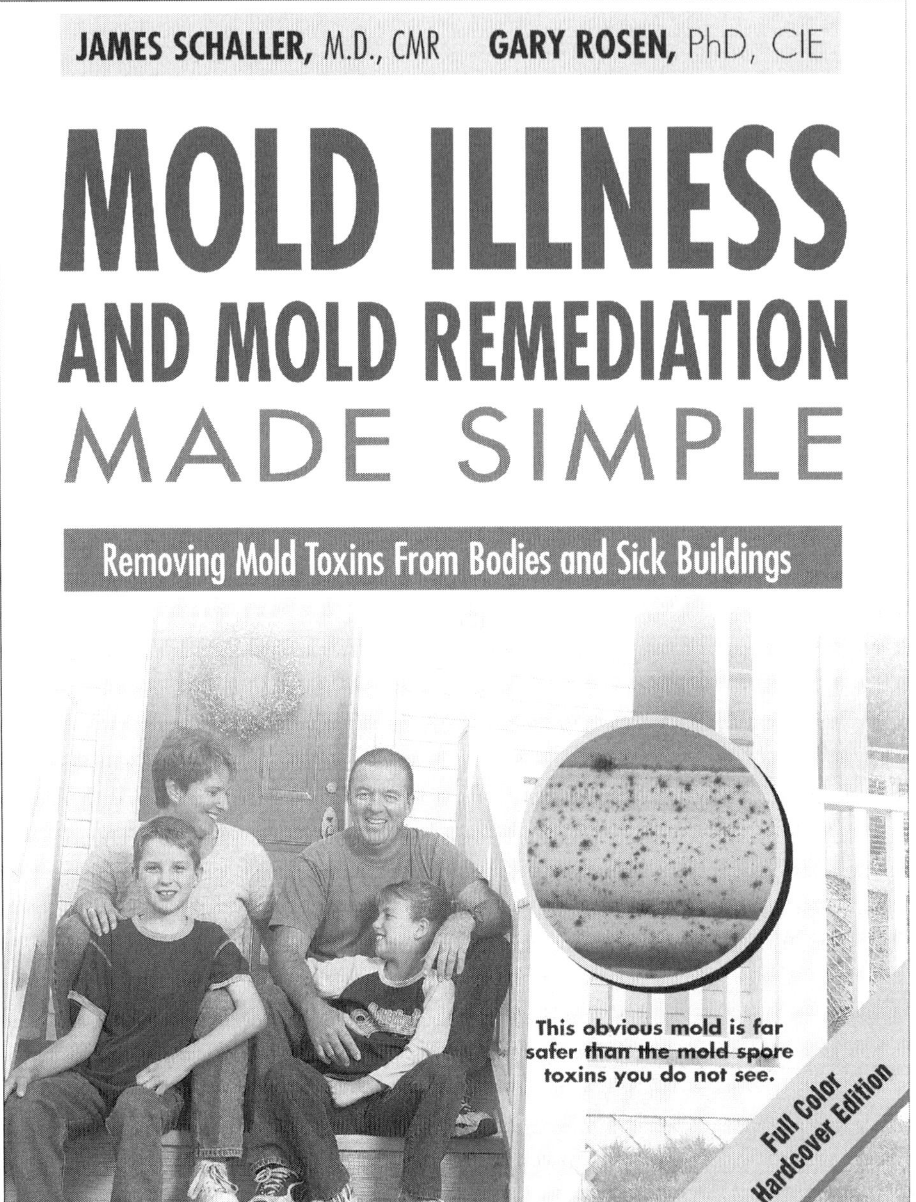

This book is helpful for people who are ill, or have trouble thinking and reading science materials. This is very practical and shows the clean-up errors made by 95% of experienced and expensive licensed mold remediators and renovation workers. Just reading ten pages from this book has shown people why they are not getting better. And this text helps you spot a poor remediators after simply reading 40 easy to understand comics. Most remediations fail and most building hygiene actions are flawed. See why fast. The six best mycotoxin binders **cannot cure you if you are *still* in a "sick" home or moldy work location.**

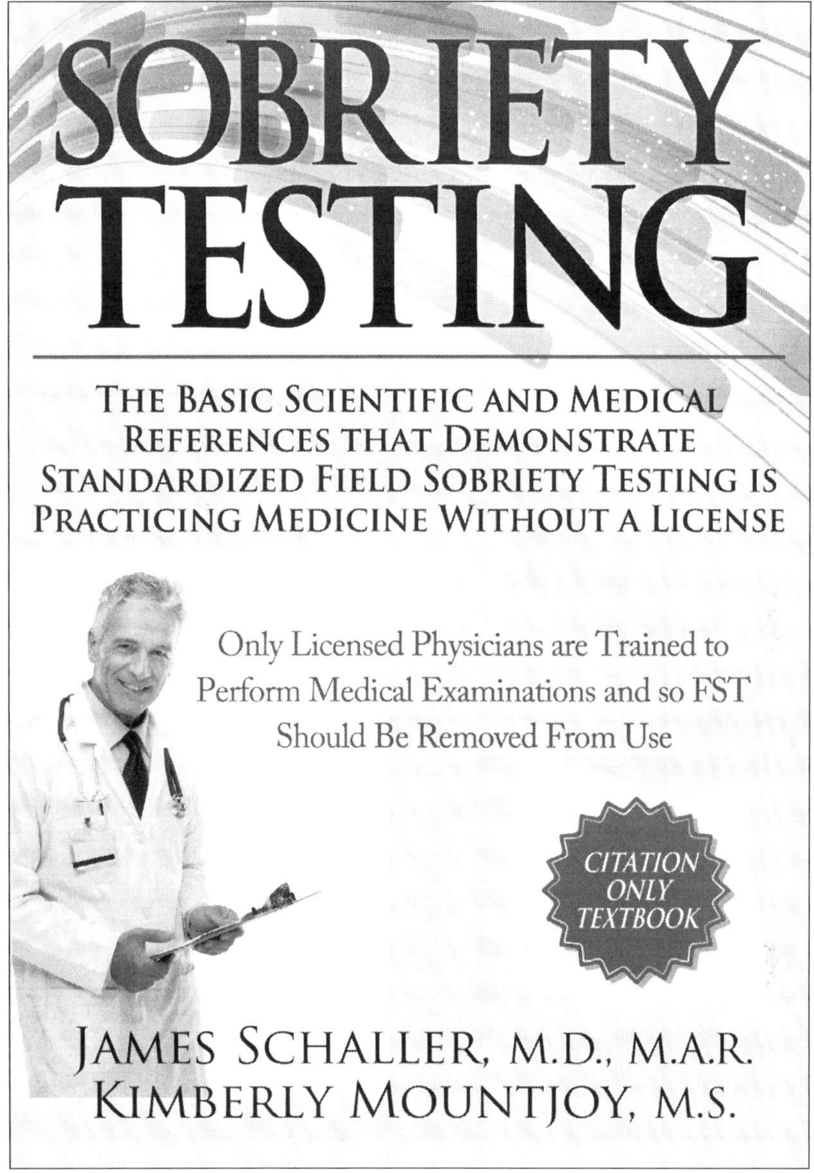

This firm book is a strong appeal for all involved in preventing impaired driving, which often causes profound disability and death, to appreciate the medical testing done on dark sidewalks or streets is a practice of advanced medical testing. FST has hundreds of routinely missed medical troubles which cause false positive tests. All civilized societies must lower the many arrests based on a lack of knowledge in human physiology and human pathology.

Further, the simplistic teaching that field sobriety testing is very easy for sober people is wrong. How many adults can walk on a balance beam a mere few feet off the ground?

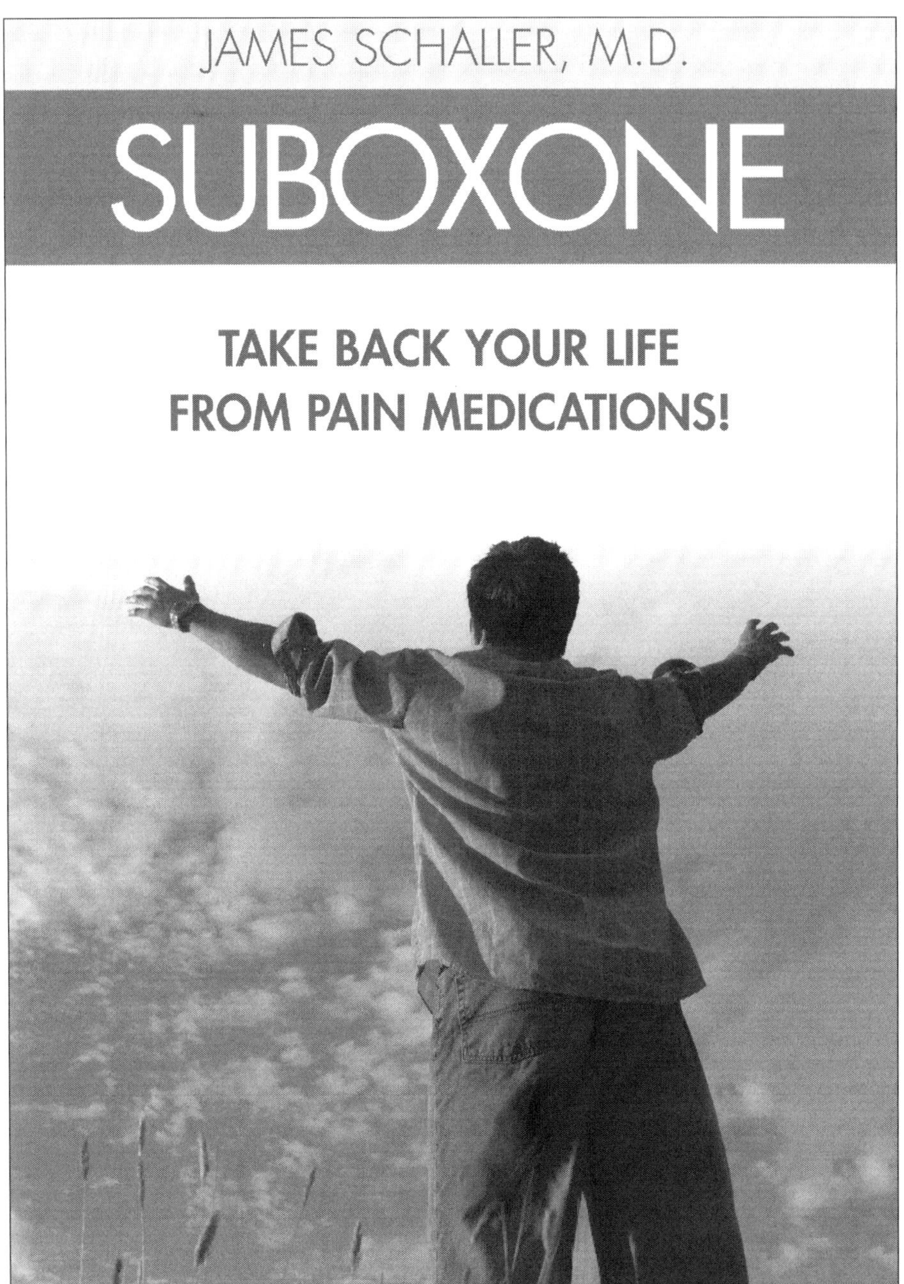

The only current, practical and advanced clinical book on this revolutionary treatment for opioid addiction and modest pain.

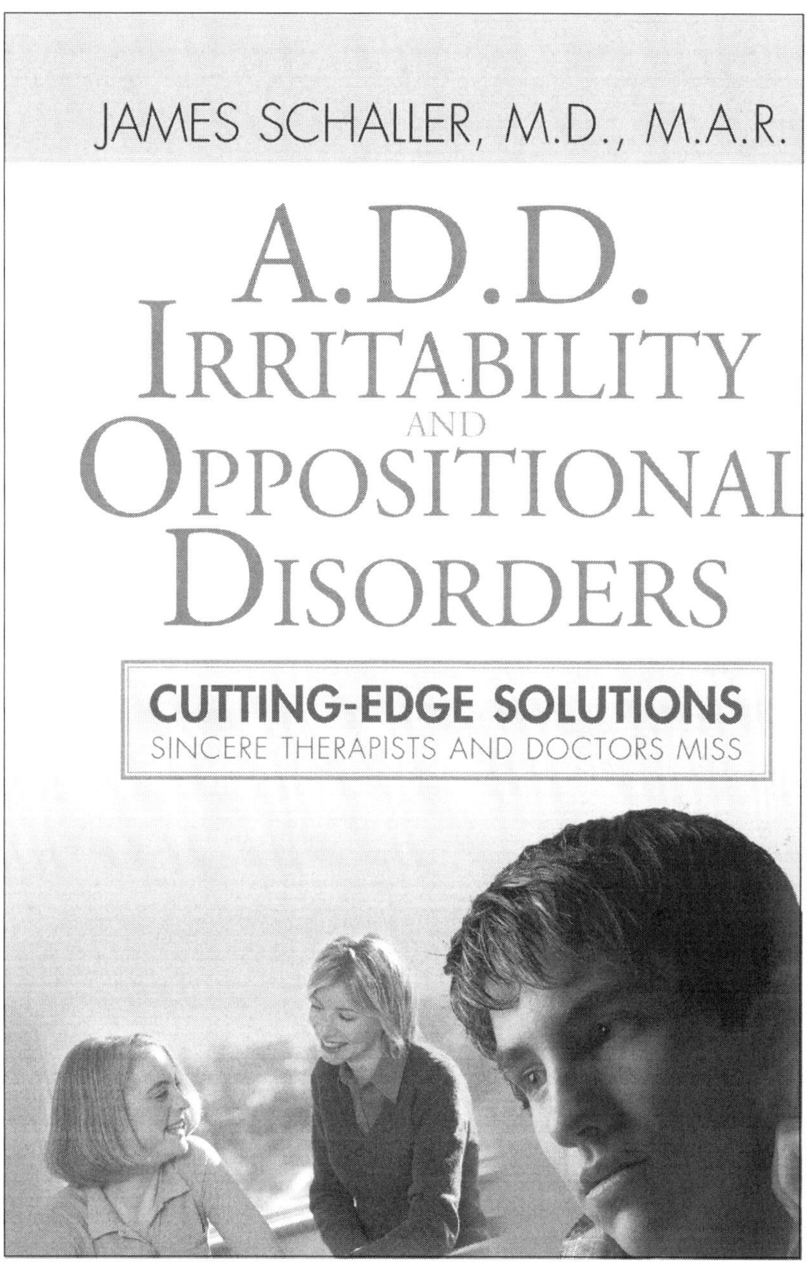

The many missed **medical and neurological** causes of poor focus and bad behaviors can no longer be ignored. This unique text advances medicine and shows how much in youth psychiatry has medical roots that are ignored or unknown even in solid child and adolescent psychiatry practices.

CHECKLISTS FOR BARTONELLA, BABESIA, AND LYME DISEASE

2012 EDITION

A "BEST DOCTOR", "PEOPLE'S CHOICE PHYSICIAN" AND "TOP DOCTOR" OFFERS HIGHLY RESEARCHED, ADVANCED DIAGNOSTIC CHECKLISTS FOR DANGEROUS EMERGING INFECTIONS

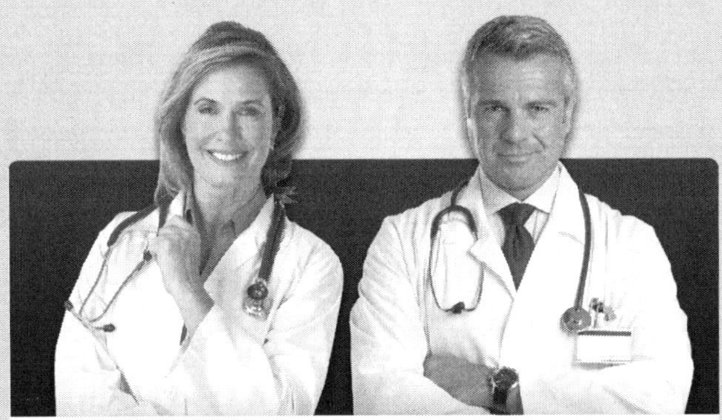

Which Physician is Going to do a Proper Exam of a Person With Bartonella, Babesia, and Lyme Disease?

The right physician is the one who is going to take the time for a very comprehensive evaluation

JAMES SCHALLER, MD, MAR & KIMBERLY MOUNTJOY, MS

The only tick and flea-borne infection diagnostic checklist book based on over 6,000 references related to Bartonella, Babesia and Lyme disease. It seeks to prevent false negative diagnosis, meaning, the advanced and expanded criteria are set to catch these three infections. This book is available from www.personalconsult.com under "free books" or from Amazon.com.

Disclaimer

Dr. Schaller is not a specialist in infectious disease medicine. He is also not a pathologist. Both of these specialties have over 2,000 diseases to treat and study. Dr. Schaller is only interested in four infections and has read and published on only these four. The medical ideas, health thoughts, health comments, products and any claims made about specific illnesses, diseases, and causes of health problems in this book are purely speculative, hypothetical, and are not meant to be authoritative in any setting. No comment or image has been evaluated by the FDA, CDC, NIH, IDSA or the AMA. Never assume any United States medical body, society, or the majority of American physicians endorse any comment in this book. No comment in this book is approved by any government agency, medical body or medical society. Nothing in this book is to be used to diagnose, treat, cure or prevent disease. The information provided in this book is for educational purposes only. It is not intended as a substitute for the advice from your physician or other health care professionals. This book is not intended to replace or adjust any information contained on, or in, any product label or packaging.

No patient should use the information in this book for the diagnosis or treatment of any health problem, or for prescription of any medication or other treatment. You should consult with a health care professional before deciding on any diagnosis, or initiating any treatment plan of any kind. Dr. Schaller does not claim to be an expert in any illness, disease or treatment. In this book, he is merely sharing one of his interests. Please do not start any diet, exercise or supplementation program, or take any type of nutrient, herb, or medication, without clear consultation with your licensed health care provider.

Babesia or Bartonella diagnosis or treatment comments and reports of possible positive or negative treatment outcomes are hypothetical. No treatment should be rejected or embraced by anyone, based on the preliminary research and study in this book.

In this book, Dr. Schaller makes no authoritative or proven claim about any diagnosis, lab testing or treatment. Dr. Schaller only offers hypothetical ideas. Dr. Schaller makes no authoritative claims about medications, nutrients, herbs or various types of alternative medicine. The ideas in this book will need to be submitted to your local expert in allopathic, osteopathic or progressive medicine, or to other licensed health care practitioners. This book is not meant to be an informal or formal guideline book that presumes to control 800,000 physicians, or the 300 million patients they serve. You are asked to let the wisdom of your health care practitioners, and your own study, be a starting point to guide treatment tailored specifically to your body. Again, Dr. Schaller makes no claim to be an expert in any aspect of medicine. He makes no claim to know more than other physicians.

Additionally, Dr. Schaller makes no claim that any statement in this book is correct.

Contacting Dr. Schaller

Should you wish to talk to Dr. Schaller he offers individualized education consults, which can be arranged by calling 239-263-0133. Please leave all your phone numbers, a working email and a fax number. These consults are typically in 15 minute units and can last as long as you wish. All that is required is the completion of a short informed consent form.

If you would like a full diagnostic consult or to see Dr. Schaller as a patient, know he treats patients from all over the USA and from outside the country. He meets with you first and then does follow-up care with you by phone.

If you would like to fly in to see Dr. Schaller, his staff are very familiar with all the closest airports, and we have special hotel discounts.

Made in the USA
San Bernardino, CA
27 May 2014